Accident and Safety Information for Teens

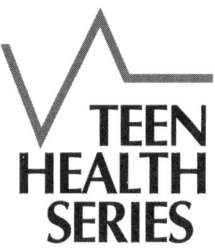

First Edition

Accident and Safety Information for Teens

Health Tips about Health Hazards, Traumatic Injuries, and Emergency Preparedness

Including Facts about Motor Vehicle Accidents, Burns, Poisoning, Firearms, Natural Disasters, National Security Threats, and More

◆

Edited by Karen Bellenir

Omnigraphics

P.O. Box 31-1640, Detroit, MI 48231

Bibliographic Note

Because this page cannot legibly accommodate all the copyright notices, the Bibliographic Note portion of the Preface constitutes an extension of the copyright notice.

Edited by Karen Bellenir

Teen Health Series
Karen Bellenir, *Managing Editor*
David A. Cooke, M.D., *Medical Consultant*
Elizabeth Collins, *Research and Permissions Coordinator*
Cherry Edwards, *Permissions Assistant*
EdIndex, Services for Publishers, *Indexers*

* * *

Omnigraphics, Inc.
Matthew P. Barbour, *Senior Vice President*
Kevin M. Hayes, *Operations Manager*

* * *

Peter E. Ruffner, *Publisher*
Copyright © 2008 Omnigraphics, Inc.
ISBN 978-0-7808-1046-4

Library of Congress Cataloging-in-Publication Data

Accident and safety information for teens : health tips about health hazards, traumatic injuries, and emergency preparedness including facts about motor vehicle accidents, burns, poisoning, firearms, natural disasters, national security threats, and more / edited by Karen Bellenir.
    p. cm. -- (Teen health series)
  Summary: "Provides basic consumer health information for teens about accident and injury prevention, disaster preparedness, and coping with emergencies. Includes index, and resource information"--Provided by publisher.
  Includes bibliographical references and index.
  ISBN 978-0-7808-1046-4 (hardcover : alk. paper) 1. Health behavior in adolescence. 2. Teenagers--Health and hygiene. 3. Health promotion. 4. Wounds and injuries--Prevention. 5. Accidents--Prevention. 6. Health education. I. Bellenir, Karen.
  RJ47.53.A33 2008
  613'.0433--dc22
                                                                  2008038383

Electronic or mechanical reproduction, including photography, recording, or any other information storage and retrieval system for the purpose of resale is strictly prohibited without permission in writing from the publisher.

The information in this publication was compiled from the sources cited and from other sources considered reliable. While every possible effort has been made to ensure reliability, the publisher will not assume liability for damages caused by inaccuracies in the data, and makes no warranty, express or implied, on the accuracy of the information contained herein.

∞

This book is printed on acid-free paper meeting the ANSI Z39.48 Standard. The infinity symbol that appears above indicates that the paper in this book meets that standard.

Printed in the United States

Table of Contents

Preface ix

Part One: Accidents Happen

Chapter 1—Dealing With An Emergency.. 3
Chapter 2—What You Should Know About 9-1-1 7
Chapter 3—First Aid Basics 17
Chapter 4—CPR: Cardiopulmonary Resuscitation 31
Chapter 5—Emergency Department Visits 35
Chapter 6—Hospitalization 43
Chapter 7—Coping With A Traumatic Experience 49

Part Two: Medical Emergencies And Traumatic Injuries

Chapter 8—Bites And Stings 57
Chapter 9—Bleeding 69
Chapter 10—Burns 75
Chapter 11—Broken Bones 87
Chapter 12—Spinal Cord Injuries 93
Chapter 13—Concussions 101
Chapter 14—Traumatic Brain Injury 107
Chapter 15—Choking 113
Chapter 16—Drug Overdose And Alcohol Poisoning 119

Part Three: Motor Vehicle Safety

Chapter 17—Teen Drivers: The Facts 127
Chapter 18—The Keys To Defensive Driving 131
Chapter 19—Questions And Answers About
                 Graduated Driver Licensing... 135
Chapter 20—Safety Belts And Teens 141
Chapter 21—What You Need To Know
                 About Air Bags 145
Chapter 22—Tire Safety.. 153
Chapter 23—Headlights And Safer Night Driving................................ 161
Chapter 24—Bad-Weather Driving Tips 169
Chapter 25—Drowsy Driving 173
Chapter 26—Young Drivers And Alcohol 179
Chapter 27—Drugged Driving 185
Chapter 28—Inattentive And Aggressive Driving.................................. 189
Chapter 29—What To Do After A Car Accident 197
Chapter 30—Motorcycle Safety 203
Chapter 31—Pedestrian Safety... 211

Part Four: Safety At Home, School, And Work

Chapter 32—How To Be Safety Savvy 219
Chapter 33—When To Call The Police 231
Chapter 34—Gun Safety 235
Chapter 35—School And School Bus Safety 239
Chapter 36—Babysitting Basics 243
Chapter 37—Fire Safety And Escape Planning...................................... 249
Chapter 38—About Fire Extinguishers 261

Chapter 39—The Dangers Of Carbon Monoxide 265

Chapter 40—Poison Prevention Tips 269

Chapter 41—Electrical And Power Outage Safety 273

Chapter 42—Lawn Maintenance Safety 281

Chapter 43—What Working Teens Need To Know
　　　　　　About Safety 289

Part Five: Outdoor And Recreation Safety

Chapter 44—Sports And Exercise Safety 297

Chapter 45—Safe Bicycling 303

Chapter 46—Water Sports And Boating 307

Chapter 47—All-Terrain Vehicles (ATVs) 315

Chapter 48—Snowmobile Safety 319

Chapter 49—Skating, Skateboarding, Skiing,
　　　　　　And Snowboarding 325

Chapter 50—Thunderstorms: Take Cover 333

Part Six: Emergency And Disaster Preparedness

Chapter 51—Making A Disaster Plan 339

Chapter 52—Sheltering In Place: What It Means 349

Chapter 53—Things To Know About Tornados,
　　　　　　Hurricanes, And Floods 353

Chapter 54—Be Prepared For Winter Storms 359

Chapter 55—Earthquakes, Volcanoes, And Wildfires:
　　　　　　What You Should Know 363

Chapter 56—Chemical Emergencies 369

Chapter 57—National Security Emergencies 381

Chapter 58—Terrorism: Preparing For The Unexpected 385

Part Seven: If You Need More Information

Chapter 59—Resources For Information About
  First Aid And Medical Emergencies 395

Chapter 60—Resources For More Information
  About Disaster Preparedness 401

Index 407

Preface

About This Book

According to statistics compiled by the National Center for Statistics and Analysis, accidents are the leading cause of death among children and youth between the ages of 8 and 20. In fact, when considered separately, various injury-related causes—traffic accidents, non-traffic related motor vehicle accidents, poisonings, drownings, falls, exposures to fire and smoke, and violence—represent five of the ten leading causes of death among those between the ages of 8 and 15 and six of the ten leading causes of death among young people between the ages of 15 and 20. In addition to the death toll, the Centers for Disease Control and Prevention estimates that injuries requiring medical attention or resulting in activity restrictions affect more than 20 million children and adolescents annually.

Accident And Safety Information For Teens provides adolescent readers with facts about what to do when accidents happen: when to call 9-1-1, what first aid steps can be taken, what to expect in the emergency department or hospital, and how to cope with the after effects of a traumatic experience. It describes serious injuries and medical emergencies, including major bleeding, burns, spinal cord injuries, brain injury, drug overdose, and alcohol poisoning. The book also provides information about motor vehicle safety, safety at home, school, and work, and outdoor and recreation-related safety. A separate section discusses emergency and disaster preparedness, including how to make a disaster plan, how to prepare for natural disasters, and what steps to take to prepare for national security emergencies. The book concludes with directories of resources for additional help and information.

How To Use This Book

This book is divided into parts and chapters. Parts focus on broad areas of interest; chapters are devoted to single topics within a part.

Part One: Accidents Happen explains what to do during emergency situations. It discusses the national emergency number, 9-1-1, and outlines steps callers can take to overcome access challenges that may arise with the use of cell phone or voice-over-the-internet technologies. It offers suggestions about being prepared to offer first aid or cardiopulmonary resuscitation (CPR), and it describes hospital and emergency department procedures. The part concludes with information about coping and adjusting after experiencing a traumatic event.

Part Two: Medical Emergencies And Traumatic Injuries describes the dangers, symptoms, and appropriate first aid steps for some of the most commonly encountered situations that may call for immediate medical assistance. These include animal bites, insect stings, bleeding, different types of burns, various kinds of fractures, head injuries, and choking. It also explains how to recognize and respond to the symptoms of alcohol poisoning, inhalant abuse, and drug overdose.

Part Three: Motor Vehicle Safety discusses car accidents—the leading cause of death for U.S. teens—and traffic safety. It describes the development of safe driving skills, the proper use of safety belts and air bags, appropriate care for tires and headlights, and the special challenges related to driving during inclement weather. Problems associated with drowsy, drunk, drugged, inattentive, and aggressive driving are also discussed, and the part concludes with chapters that address the special concerns of motorcyclists and pedestrians.

Part Four: Safety At Home, School, And Work helps readers become aware of risks they may face in everyday settings. It describes steps teens can take to protect themselves as they encounter new or different social situations, assume more responsibilities, and move into the work force.

Part Five: Outdoor And Recreation Safety includes sports injury prevention tips and offers suggestions for avoiding hazards associated with bicycling, swimming, boating, driving all-terrain vehicles, snowmobiling, skating, skateboarding, skiing, and snowboarding. It also describes taking appropriate precautions and finding shelter if a thunderstorm develops.

Part Six: Emergency And Disaster Preparedness describes the process of planning ahead for natural disasters and national security emergencies. It offers check lists of emergency supplies and discusses what to expect in the event of a tornado, hurricane, flood, winter storm, earthquake, volcano, wildfire, or other incident associated with the untamed aspect of nature. It also explains steps that can be taken to be ready to respond to man-made disasters, such as chemical accidents and acts of terrorism.

Part Seven: If You Need More Information includes directories of resources for additional facts about first aid, medical emergencies, and disaster preparedness.

Bibliographic Note

This volume contains documents and excerpts from publications issued by the following federal government agencies: Centers for Disease Control and Prevention; Federal Emergency Management Agency; Federal Highway Administration; National Highway Traffic Safety Administration; National Institute for Occupational Safety and Health; National Institute of Neurological Disorders and Stroke; National Institute on Alcohol Abuse and Alcoholism; National Institute on Drug Abuse; National Women's Health Information Center; U.S. Coast Guard; U.S. Department of Homeland Security; U.S. Department of Justice; U.S. Department of Labor; and the U.S. Fire Administration.

In addition, this volume contains copyrighted documents and articles produced by the following organizations and individuals: A.D.A.M., Inc.; AAA Foundation for Traffic Safety; American Academy of Family Physicians; American National Red Cross; Children, Youth and Women's Health Services, Government of South Australia; City of Miami, Department of Fire-Rescue; Hanford Fire Department; David J. Hanson, Ph.D.; Home Safety Council; HowStuffWorks.com; Insurance Institute for Highway Safety, Highway Loss Data Institute; International Snowmobile Manufacturers Association; Muscogee (Creek) Nation Emergency Management; National Crime Prevention Council; National Emergency Number Association; National Safety Council; National Sleep Foundation; Nemours Foundation; New Zealand Dermatological Society; NHS Direct Online (Scotland); Safe Kids Worldwide; Shriners Hospitals for Children; Texas AgriLife Extension Service; and ThinkFirst National Injury Prevention Foundation.

Full citation information is provided on the first page of each chapter. Every effort has been made to secure all necessary rights to reprint the copyrighted material. If any omissions have been made, please contact Omnigraphics to make corrections for future editions.

The photograph on the front cover is from Mary Gascho/iStockphoto.

Acknowledgements

In addition to the organizations listed above, special thanks are due to research and permissions coordinator, Liz Collins; permissions assistant, Cherry Stockdale; editorial assistants, Elizabeth Bellenir and Nicole Salerno; and prepress technician, Stephen G. Wesley.

About the *Teen Health Series*

At the request of librarians serving today's young adults, the *Teen Health Series* was developed as a specially focused set of volumes within Omnigraphics' *Health Reference Series*. Each volume deals comprehensively with a topic selected according to the needs and interests of people in middle school and high school.

Teens seeking preventive guidance, information about disease warning signs, medical statistics, and risk factors for health problems will find answers to their questions in the *Teen Health Series*. The *Series*, however, is not intended to serve as a tool for diagnosing illness, in prescribing treatments, or as a substitute for the physician/patient relationship. All people concerned about medical symptoms or the possibility of disease are encouraged to seek professional care from an appropriate health care provider.

If there is a topic you would like to see addressed in a future volume of the *Teen Health Series*, please write to:

Editor
Teen Health Series
Omnigraphics, Inc.
P.O. Box 31-1640
Detroit, MI 48231

Locating Information within the *Teen Health Series*

The *Teen Health Series* contains a wealth of information about a wide variety of medical topics. As the Series continues to grow in size and scope, locating the precise information needed by a specific student may become more challenging. To address this concern, information about books within the *Teen Health Series* is included in *A Contents Guide to the Health Reference Series*. The *Contents Guide* presents an extensive list of more than 14,000 diseases, treatments, and other topics of general interest compiled from the Tables of Contents and major index headings from the books of the *Teen Health Series* and *Health Reference Series*. To access *A Contents Guide to the Health Reference Series*, visit www.healthreferenceseries.com.

Our Advisory Board

We would like to thank the following advisory board members for providing guidance to the development of this Series:

Dr. Lynda Baker, Associate Professor of Library and Information Science, Wayne State University, Detroit, MI

Nancy Bulgarelli, William Beaumont Hospital Library, Royal Oak, MI

Karen Imarisio, Bloomfield Township Public Library, Bloomfield Township, MI

Karen Morgan, Mardigian Library, University of Michigan-Dearborn, Dearborn, MI

Rosemary Orlando, St. Clair Shores Public Library, St. Clair Shores, MI

Medical Consultant

Medical consultation services are provided to the *Teen Health Series* editors by David A. Cooke, M.D. Dr. Cooke is a graduate of Brandeis University, and he received his M.D. degree from the University of Michigan. He completed residency training at the University of Wisconsin Hospital and Clinics. He is board-certified in internal medicine. Dr. Cooke currently works as part of the University of Michigan Health System and practices in Ann Arbor, MI. In his free time, he enjoys writing, science fiction, and spending time with his family.

Part One
Accidents Happen

Chapter 1

Dealing With An Emergency

Emergencies happen when we least expect them, and they require fast thinking and action. But different emergencies call for different approaches. Here are some things to know so you'll be prepared.

When To Call 911

A 911 emergency is a situation in which someone needs immediate help because he or she is injured or in immediate danger. So if you've had a car accident and someone is hurt, obviously you'll call 911. But if your car just broke down and you need a tow truck, you'll need to call a towing service (or, better still, your parents).

Call 911 if there's a fire, if someone has had an accident, or if you see a crime being committed. Don't hesitate to call 911 if a friend has taken drugs or done something else that's life threatening. You may be afraid you'll get your friend in trouble, but calling could mean the difference between life and death.

When you call 911, the emergency dispatch operator will probably ask what, where, and who questions such as:

About This Chapter: "Dealing With An Emergency," May 2005, reprinted with permission from www.kidshealth.org. Copyright © 2005 The Nemours Foundation. This information was provided by KidsHealth, one of the largest resources online for medically reviewed health information written for parents, kids, and teens. For more articles like this one, visit www.KidsHealth.org, or www.TeensHealth.org.

- "What is the emergency?" or "What happened?"
- "Where are you?" or "Where do you live?"
- "Who needs help?" or "Who is with you?"

Although you may feel a sense of panic when faced with an emergency, try your best to stay in control. The operator needs the answers to specific questions to decide what type of emergency workers should be sent and where to send them. Give the operator all the relevant information you can about what the emergency is and how it happened. If someone is unconscious or has stopped breathing, the 911 operator may give you instructions for immediate help that you can provide, such as administering CPR (cardiopulmonary resuscitation) or clearing the person's breathing passage.

You know that you need to stay calm and speak slowly and clearly so that the 911 operator can understand you. But did you know you should stay on the phone and not hang up until the operator tells you it is OK? That way, you can be sure that the operator has all the information that's needed to get help to you fast. It's easy to assume that operators can trace where a call is coming from, but that's not always the case.

If you dial 911 by mistake—you hit the wrong button on your phone, for example—don't just hang up. In areas where dispatchers can trace the call, you could find a fire truck or police car in your driveway. Tell the operator what happened so that he or she knows that there is no real emergency.

> ♣ **It's A Fact!!**
> **When Not To Call 911**
>
> Emergency dispatchers stress that you should never call 911 for information, for your pets, or to pay a traffic ticket. Dialing 911 as a prank is considered a crime in many places. It's that strict because whenever a 911 operator has to take a non-emergency call, it could delay getting emergency services to someone who really needs them.

Dealing With An Emergency

If you're ever in doubt and no one is around to ask, it's better to call 911 and let the operator decide if it's a real emergency than to take the chance that someone who needs help doesn't get it quickly.

Safety Tips

In situations where you're in charge, such as babysitting or caring for someone with a health condition, you need to be prepared in advance for emergencies. Here are some things you can do so you can respond quickly if something happens:

- Make sure there's a list of emergency numbers near each telephone in the house. Most areas in the United States are covered by 911 service. But if you live somewhere that does not have 911 service, have numbers for the police department, the fire department, and emergency medical services handy. If you have a cell phone, it's a good idea to program important numbers into your phone.

- Keep on hand numbers for adults you should call. If you're babysitting, make sure you have the number and location where the child's parents will be and, if possible, a cell phone or pager number. If it's a true emergency—a child you're caring for has stopped breathing, for example—always call 911 first and then call the parent.

- If you're looking after someone with a health condition, know when the person needs to take any medications—particularly medicines for breathing or heart problems. Have the person's insurance information on hand in case you need to rush to the hospital. It's a good idea to keep all this information written down near the phone so that you can find it quickly if you need it.

- Make sure the home or building you're in has working smoke alarms.

- Make sure your family or the family you're caring for has a fire escape plan and that children know their outdoor meeting point in case of an emergency.

- Take a first-aid class to learn CPR so you'll be prepared to help someone in an emergency.

- Make sure the poison control center phone number is handy. Some areas have toll-free numbers available.
- Keep a first-aid kit in the house and know how to use it.

When Someone's Been Hurt

If someone's been in an accident and is unconscious, don't try to move the person—he or she may have a neck or spine injury. Call 911 or get help first (or have someone else get help while you take care of the injured person). If the person is bleeding, put pressure on the wound with a cloth or piece of clothing to slow the blood flow. Don't try to clean the wound, though, as it may do more damage. Wait with the person until help arrives.

Don't rush to help someone if the area isn't safe—if the victim is in the middle of a road, for example, or if you have to put yourself in danger to get to him or her. Make sure it's safe before you try to get to the person and help.

If a person who's been injured is conscious, he or she may still be at risk of internal injury or concussion. In some accidents, people seem fine at first but end up having internal injuries. So it's a good idea to call 911 or take the person to the emergency department to get checked out. If someone is disoriented, feels sick, or has a headache, he or she may have a concussion or other head injury.

✔ **Quick Tip**

Natural Disasters

If you live in an area prone to natural disasters, such as tornadoes or earthquakes, know what to do in an emergency. You can find out what to do in different situations by visiting the Centers for Disease Control and Prevention's Emergency Preparedness and Response site (available online at http://emergency.cdc.gov).

If the weather is bad, listen to the radio or TV so you can be aware of any plans to evacuate your area.

Dealing with an emergency can be scary for anyone. You can take away some of the fear factor by making sure you and other people in your house are prepared and know what to do if an emergency does come up.

Chapter 2

What You Should Know About 9-1-1

9-1-1 General Information

What is 9-1-1?

Nine-one-one is the number most people in the U.S. and some in international countries call to get help in a police, fire, or medical emergency. In some places, you may be able to be connected with Poison Control by calling 9-1-1, but you should check with local officials in your area to make sure. A 9-1-1 call goes over dedicated phone lines to the 9-1-1 answering point closest to the caller, and trained personnel then send the emergency help needed.

What is enhanced 9-1-1?

Enhanced 9-1-1, or E9-1-1, is a system which routes an emergency call to the 9-1-1 center closest to the caller, and automatically displays the caller's phone number and address. The 9-1-1 call taker will typically ask the caller to verify the information, which appears on his or her computer screen. In most areas, phone number and location information is not yet available for 9-1-1 calls made from a cellular/wireless phone.

About This Chapter: This chapter includes "9-1-1 General Information," "Wireless 9-1-1 Overview," and "Frequently Asked Questions," © 2006 National Emergency Number Association (www.nena.org and www.911voip.org); reprinted with permission.

When should you use 9-1-1?

Nine-one-one is only to be used in emergency situations. An emergency is any situation that requires immediate assistance from the police/sheriff, the fire department, or an ambulance. If you are ever in doubt of whether a situation is an emergency you should call 9-1-1. It's better to be safe and let the 9-1-1 call taker determine if you need emergency assistance.

Do not call 9-1-1:

- for information;
- for directory assistance;
- when you're bored and just want to talk;
- for paying tickets;
- for your pet; or
- as a prank.

> ♣ **It's A Fact!!**
> **Who pays for 9-1-1?**
>
> Each household or business pays a small monthly fee for 9-1-1 service on each telephone line that appears on their phone bill. There is no per-call charge for calling 9-1-1. However, EMS/ambulances dispatched through 9-1-1 may charge for taking someone to the hospital; this is a separate ambulance charge, not a 9-1-1 charge.
>
> Source: "9-1-1 General Information," © 2006 National Emergency Number Association.

If you call 9-1-1 by mistake, do not hang up. Tell the call taker what happened so they know there really isn't an emergency.

What about 9-1-1 prank calls?

It's a prank call when someone calls 9-1-1 for a joke or calls 9-1-1 and hangs up. Prank calls not only waste time and money, but can also be dangerous. If 9-1-1 lines or call takers are busy with prank calls, someone with a real emergency may not be able to get the help they need. In most places, it's against the law to make prank 9-1-1 calls.

What You Should Know About 9-1-1

How do you make a 9-1-1 call?

- In an emergency, dial 9-1-1 on your phone. It's a free call. You can use any kind of phone: push button, rotary, cellular/wireless, cordless, or pay phone. (With some pay phones, you may need coins to get a dial tone; with many wireless phones, enhanced 9-1-1 does not yet work.)
- Stay calm and state your emergency.
- Speak loudly and clearly. Give the 9-1-1 call taker your name, phone number and the address where help is needed.
- Answer the call taker's questions. Stay on the telephone if it's safe to do so, and don't hang up until the call taker tells you to.

What if a 9-1-1 caller doesn't speak English?

When necessary, a 9-1-1 call taker can add an interpreter from an outside service to the line. A non-English speaking caller may hear a short conversation in English and some clicking sounds as the interpreter is added to the line.

What if a 9-1-1 caller is deaf or hearing/speech impaired?

Communications centers that answer 9-1-1 calls have special text telephones for responding to 9-1-1 calls from deaf or hearing/speech impaired callers. If a caller uses a TTY/TDD, the caller should:

- Stay calm, place the phone receiver in the TTY, dial 9-1-1.
- After the call is answered, press the TTY keys several times. This may help shorten the time necessary to respond to the call.
- Give the call taker time to connect their TTY. If necessary, press the TTY keys again. The 9-1-1 call taker should answer and type "GA" for Go Ahead.
- Tell what is needed—police, fire department, or ambulance. Give your name, phone number, and the address where help is needed.
- Stay on the telephone if it is safe. Answer the call taker's questions.

If a deaf or hearing/speech impaired caller doesn't have a TTY/TDD, the caller should call 9-1-1 and don't hang up. Not hanging up leaves the line open. With most 9-1-1 calls, the caller's address is displayed on the call taker's screen and help will be sent.

Wireless 9-1-1 Overview

What Is Wireless 9-1-1?

In most areas of North America, citizens have basic or enhanced 9-1-1 service from their landline, or wireline, phones in their homes or workplaces. Basic 9-1-1 means that when the three-digit number is dialed, a call taker/dispatcher in the local public safety answering point (PSAP), or 9-1-1 center, answers the call. The emergency and its location are communicated by voice between the caller and the call taker. In areas serviced by enhanced 9-1-1, the local 9-1-1 center has equipment and database information that allow the call taker to see the caller's phone number and address on a display. This lets them quickly dispatch emergency help, even if the caller is unable to communicate where they are or what the emergency is.

However, when 9-1-1 calls are made from wireless phones, the call may not be routed to the closest 9-1-1 center, and the call taker doesn't receive the callback phone number or the location of the caller. This presents life-threatening problems due to lost response time, if callers are unable to speak or don't know where they are, or if they don't know their wireless phone callback number and the call is dropped.

Three Phases Of Wireless 9-1-1

There are three phases that are referred to in implementing wireless 9-1-1. The most basic of these, sometimes called Wireless Phase 0, simply means that when you dial 9-1-1 from your cell phone a call taker at a public safety answering point (PSAP) answers. The call taker may be at a state highway patrol PSAP, at a city or county PSAP up to hundreds of miles away, or at a local PSAP, depending on how the wireless 9-1-1 call is routed.

Wireless Phase I is the first step in providing better emergency response service to wireless 9-1-1 callers. When Phase I has been implemented, a wireless 9-1-1 call will come into the PSAP with the wireless phone call back number. This is important in the event the cell phone call is dropped,

What You Should Know About 9-1-1

and may even allow PSAP employees to work with the wireless company to identify the wireless subscriber. However, Phase I still doesn't help call takers locate emergency victims or callers.

To locate wireless 9-1-1 callers, Phase II must have been implemented in the area by local 9-1-1 systems and wireless carriers. Phase II allows call takers to receive both the caller's wireless phone number and their location information.

Wireless 9-1-1 Requirements

Phase 0: Required by basic 911 rules (according to the Federal Communications Commission, FCC). Wireless 9-1-1 calls are to be transmitted to a PSAP regardless of whether being placed by a wireless service subscriber or non-subscriber.

Phase I: April 1, 1998 or within six months of being requested by the PSAP, whichever comes later.

Phase II: Originally, October 1, 2001. Specific requirements differ for network-based and handset-based solutions.

A Critical Public Safety Issue

"[Wireless 9-1-1] is rapidly becoming a critical public safety issue affecting all Americans," said W. Mark Adams, NENA's Executive Director, in a June 1999 NENA press release. "In the 16 years since cell phones were introduced, 9-1-1 operators have not been able to automatically receive the location or even the phone number of people calling from a wireless phone."

The industry set forth to educate itself, our legislators, and our public of the critical need for wireless 9-1-1 service. After having been the topic of discussion in 9-1-1 for several years, wireless 9-1-1 service is finally becoming a reality. With a sturdy infrastructure and the technology necessary to support wireless 9-1-1 service, members of each state's public safety community have worked—or are working—tirelessly to pass the legislation necessary to fund this valuable, necessary, and overdue component to the public safety system.

Now, with legislation, funding, and the technology in hand or on the way, the challenge is being met and our wireless telephone users can be confident that—in the future—help will indeed be on the way when they dial 9-1-1 from a cell phone.

Frequently Asked Questions About Internet Phone Service

Can I dial 9-1-1 from my voice over internet protocol (VoIP) phone?

You can reach emergency assistance by dialing 9-1-1 on most VoIP phones. However, there are important differences between some VoIP 9-1-1 emergency dialing and traditional 9-1-1 service from a standard phone. It is important to familiarize yourself with these differences. Often the 9-1-1 call taker will not have a display of the number you called from or your location. In addition, your call may arrive at a remote private call center or a non-emergency line, without a display of your location.

How do I know what level of 9-1-1 service I have with my VoIP phone?

You need to research the features of your VoIP service as it pertains to emergency dialing by accessing the service provider's website. Search provider's websites for "emergency calling". Once you are aware of the 9-1-1 limitations, you need to notify all potential users of the phone (spouse, children, babysitters, etc.).

How is my 9-1-1 call routed to the correct location?

When you sign up for VoIP you must register your location. In order for 9-1-1 emergency dialing to work properly, the service address of file for you must correspond to the physical location of your VoIP phone. This will enable your VoIP service provider to identify your 9-1-1 call center. You cannot specify a P.O. Box.

What if my 9-1-1 call is misrouted to the incorrect 9-1-1 answering point?

If your VoIP 9-1-1 call is not routed to the correct 9-1-1 call center, you should tell the call taker the city, county, and state where you need help. The call taker can attempt to transfer your emergency call to the correct call center.

What You Should Know About 9-1-1

> ### ♣ It's A Fact!!
> ### Wireless Statistics
>
> In our increasingly wireless society, more and more of the mobile public is dialing 9-1-1 every day—about 86 million people were subscribers of wireless telephone service in 1999, according to the Cellular Telephone Industry Association (CTIA). In addition, CTIA estimates that nearly 46,000 Americans become wireless subscribers every day.
>
> It is estimated that of the 150 million calls that were made to 9-1-1 in 2000, 45 million of them were made by wireless telephone users—that's 30 percent. This is a ten-fold increase from nearly 4.3 million wireless 9-1-1 calls just 10 years ago, and the number will more than double to 100 million calls in the next five years. It is anticipated that by 2005, the majority of 9-1-1 calls will have been from wireless callers.
>
> Beginning in 2006, statistical information on wireless 9-1-1 will be more exact and readily available within the National Emergency Number Association's (NENA) Report Card to the Nation project. In this first ever nation-wide survey of the industry, NENA will track a variety of 9-1-1 system information including wireline and wireless call statistics, 9-1-1 service levels, legislation, equipment, staffing information, and more.
>
> Frightening statistics about wireless calls to 9-1-1, like those stated above, and the actions of industries tangential to 9-1-1 have brought us together to develop solutions that will ultimately work best for the citizens we serve.
>
> Source: "Wireless 9-1-1 Overview," © 2006 National Emergency Number Association.

It is a good idea to know what police, fire, or sheriff's department is responsible for your 9-1-1 calls and have their 10-digit phone number on hand to provide the call taker.

Can I call 9-1-1 from my VoIP phone when I'm traveling?

Your VoIP provider may offer the ability to travel with, or move your VoIP service to take advantage of any location with broadband internet access. Your VoIP service provider should offer at least one way to update your registered location. However, the time it takes to update or make

> ♣ **It's A Fact!!**
> **Does 9-1-1 know where I am when calling from my VoIP phone?**
>
> It depends. The first information you will need to provide or verify for the 9-1-1 call taker is your location, name, and telephone number, especially if the emergency service personnel does not have this information available automatically. When this occurs, your call goes to a remote private call center or non-emergency line at the 9-1-1 center, which is different from how traditional 9-1-1 calls are routed to an emergency call center.
>
> Source: "Frequently Asked Questions," © 2006 National Emergency Number Association.

any changes to your registered location varies greatly. If you relocate your VoIP phone on a temporary basis, such as taking it with you when you go on a trip, don't use it to get emergency help. Use another telephone to dial 9-1-1.

What if my 9-1-1 call is disconnected or cut off?

Unlike traditional 9-1-1 service, the 9-1-1 call taker may not be able to call you back if you are disconnected. They may not have access to your phone number. If you are disconnected, hang up and dial 9-1-1 again.

Do service outages affect my ability to call 9-1-1?

They may. Just as your regular cordless phone will not work without power, your VoIP phone may not work without power either. As a result, you may be unable to make any calls, including those to 9-1-1 during an electrical power outage.

Similarly, you may not be able to make 9-1-1 calls from your VoIP phone if your broadband or cable service provider has an outage or if any other service disruptions keep you from being able to make any outbound call.

What You Should Know About 9-1-1   15

Do I need to notify someone if I move?

Yes. When you move, you must update your registered location on your service provider's website. It may take several days to update your record.

Should I keep my traditional phone line after I subscribe to VoIP service?

Yes. 9-1-1 industry leaders recommend that you keep your traditional phone line in addition to your VoIP phone service in order to successfully access 9-1-1 services and to have telephone access during a power outage.

Do I need to tell anyone in my family that I have changed our phone service?

Yes. It is very important that all persons that live in your home understand the differences in emergency calling with your new VoIP service. Children and babysitters always need to be educated on how to call 9-1-1 in an emergency. You might want to post your phone number and address by the phone for easy access.

Will my home/business security monitoring service work with my VoIP service?

It might, but it might not. Check with your VoIP service provider to see if they support analog modem traffic such as burglar alarms, fax machines, and DVRs (digital video recorders), such as Tivo.

♣ It's A Fact!!
Can I make a 9-1-1 test call from my VoIP phone?

It depends. Before doing so, please contact your 9-1-1 call center on their non-emergency line. Confirm that you are in their 9-1-1 jurisdiction and then ask if you can place a test 9-1-1 call. Many 9-1-1 call centers will comply with this request as long as they are not too busy with other emergency calls at the time. They may ask you to place your test call at a certain time.

Source: "Frequently Asked Questions," © 2006 National Emergency Number Association.

Chapter 3
First Aid Basics

Below you will find some basic guidelines to help you help yourself and others during a medical crisis. The information presented here is to be used as an introduction to first aid. It is not intended as a substitute for professional medical advice and care, treatment by trained emergency personnel, or first aid and CPR (cardiopulmonary resuscitation) training. If you are in a life- or limb-threatening emergency, call for medical help immediately.

Emergency Warning Signs

Look for these emergency warning signs that indicate a person could suffer major harm or die without immediate care. Call 911 immediately if one or more of these signs are present.

- Prolonged chest pain (lasting two or more minutes)
- Uncontrolled bleeding
- Difficulty breathing or shortness of breath
- Choking or vomiting blood
- Severe pain

About This Chapter: "Basic First Aid Guidelines," reprinted with permission from Muscogee (Creek) Nation Emergency Management; © Muscogee (Creek) Nation; Emergency Management. This document is available online at http://www.muscogeenation-nsn.gov/emer%20mgmt/CPRFirst%20Aid%20Guidlines1.pdf; accessed February 18, 2008.

- A weak or nonexistent heartbeat when checking for a pulse on the neck alongside the Adam's apple
- Sudden weakness, change in vision, or dizziness
- Persistent vomiting or diarrhea
- Confusion or difficulty arousing

Action

- Remain calm, be aware of your surroundings, and closely evaluate the scene to protect yourself and others from further injury.
- Do not move a critically injured person unless instructed by emergency medical professionals.
- Do not try to drive someone who is critically ill or injured to a hospital unless there is no way to summon emergency help.
- Call 911 or ask someone else to call:
    - if you think there is a medical emergency, or
    - if the crisis could get worse left untreated or not treated properly.
- Listen carefully to the 911 dispatcher's questions. Answer them calmly and quickly.
- Remain on the line until the dispatcher tells you it's okay to hang up.
- Ask someone to wait outside to meet emergency personnel if it is safe to do so.
- Paramedics may want to know a brief summary of the circumstances that caused the emergency. Remain calm and cooperative as they gather information.

Preparing For An Emergency

There are some things you can do to help prepare for emergencies at home:

- Create first aid kits for your home and cars. Each kit should include adhesive bandages, sterile gauze pads and tape, an elastic (ACE) bandage, a

First Aid Basics

triangular bandage to fashion slings, antiseptic wipes, tweezers, scissors, antibiotic ointment, calamine and hydrocortisone lotions, syrup of ipecac, cold packs, and a first-aid manual. You can add other items—such as bottled water or a thermometer—to your kits. Be sure to check your kit regularly to replace expired or depleted supplies.

- Organize medical information—including major diseases or disorders, lists of medication names and dosages, blood type, and a summary of allergies—for each member of your family.

♣ It's A Fact!!
First Aid Kit

Your basic first aid kit should contain the following items:

- An antiseptic (Betadine)
- Ice bag or cold pack
- Antibiotic spray or ointment
- Scissors with rounded ends
- Adhesive bandages (various sizes)
- Tweezers
- Adhesive tape (1½" to 1" wide)
- Thermometer
- Sterile gauze pads
- Aspirin
- Hydrocortisone cream or calamine lotion (to relieve minor itching)
- Syrup of ipecac (for swallowed poisons: use as directed by the Poison Control Center)

Caution: Be sure that all supplies are kept out of the reach of young children.

Source: Excerpted from an undated document accessed February 18, 2008: "Basic First Aid Procedures," © City of Miami Department of Fire-Rescue (www.ci.miami.fl.us/Fire). Reprinted with permission.

- Review safety procedures and eliminate hazards.
- Take classes to learn first aid and CPR.

Bleeding

Bleeding can involve minor cuts and scrapes or may be caused by major puncture wounds or injuries. Most injuries can be treated at home or in an urgent care facility, but if someone is bleeding uncontrollably, call 911.

Classifications Of Bleeding

- **Capillary:** Small cuts and scrapes open the capillaries, and bleeding occurs. The bleeding is slow and generally clots within a matter of minutes.
- **Venous:** Deep cuts may open a vein that carries blood back to the heart. The blood is dark in color and flows slowly. Pressure will usually stop this type of injury.
- **Arterial:** Injuries that cause arterial bleeding are very serious and require immediate medical attention. Blood from an arterial bleed is bright red and spurts out in rhythm with the heart pumping. Applying pressure will not stop the bleeding. It is important to get help immediately!

Serious Wounds

If blood is gushing or spurting from the wound, call for emergency help. If too much blood is lost, it can result in unconsciousness, shock, or even death. Until emergency help arrives:

- Make sure the victim is lying down. Position his head lower than the rest of his body, or elevate his legs.
- Watch for indications of shock (including lack of focus, cold and clammy hands, change in speech, and inability to remember things) or difficulty breathing.
- Clean out debris or dirt from the injury.
- Don't remove any objects stuck deep inside the victim.

First Aid Basics 21

- Using a clean cloth, towel, piece of clothing, or your hand, apply pressure to the wound. Maintain pressure for at least 10 minutes.
- If bleeding seeps through the material you're using, don't remove it, simply add more on top. If direct pressure doesn't stop the bleeding, you may need to put pressure on the artery which supplies blood to the affected area.
- Elevate the site of the injury.
- Leave the bandage in place and get emergency help immediately!

Minor Wounds

The kinds of cuts and scrapes you get everyday don't require a trip to the emergency room, but you need to make sure the wound is taken care of to prevent infection.

- When cuts or scrapes occur, you first need to stop the bleeding. An injury which does not require emergency treatment will quit bleeding within a few minutes. If bleeding doesn't stop on its own, apply pressure with a gauze pad or clean cloth. If bleeding continues to flow or spurt, you may need to get medical attention.
- Clean the wound. Wash the affected area with mild soap and water. If there is any material embedded in the injury that does not come loose during cleaning, consult a physician. Once the wound is clean, pat the area dry with a clean cloth. Unless the injury is to the face, apply antiseptic or antibiotic cream. You can cover the injury with a bandage.
- If the injury is deep or has jagged edges, it may require stitches to heal properly and minimize scarring. Consult a physician if you are not sure.
- Keep the injury area clean and change the bandage daily.
- If the area of the injury becomes swollen, red, or begins oozing fluids, you need to be evaluated by a physician.

Choking

In adults, choking is usually caused by food lodged in the throat or windpipe. Victims will instinctively grab at the throat and may panic, wheeze, or gasp for breath.

If a person can cough and speak and has normal skin color, he or she is getting air and is not choking. Encourage the person to continue coughing to resolve the partial blockage. Do not hit him on the back or try to give water.

If the person cannot cough or speak, the windpipe is blocked and he is choking and needs emergency help.

The Heimlich Maneuver

The Heimlich maneuver is an abdominal thrust that forces air up and out with enough force to clear the airway. The procedure can be used on adults and children one year and older. To perform the Heimlich maneuver:

- Stand behind the victim and wrap your arms around his waist, bending him slightly forward.

- Place a fist just above the victim's navel. Cover your fist with the other hand and begin squeezing with quick, hard thrusts into the abdomen inward and upward.

- Continue until the obstruction is cleared and the person is able to breathe.

The Heimlich maneuver can be adapted to other circumstances, such as with babies younger than one year, pregnant or obese people, or with a person who has lost consciousness.

- For obese and pregnant victims, put your hands at the base of their breastbones, right where the lowest ribs join together.

- For infants, hold the baby face down on your forearm. Thump the baby on the back five times. If he does not begin breathing, turn him over with the head positioned lower than the body. Using two fingers, compress his breastbone five times.

- The procedure can be done on yourself if you are choking and alone. Give yourself abdominal thrusts, or stand over the back of a chair or counter and press against it hard to dislodge the airway obstruction.

Choking is an emergency. Call for help. Don't try to drive the victim to a hospital!

First Aid Basics

Broken Bones

A broken bone is also called a fracture. This type of injury is accompanied by intense pain, difficulty or inability to move the injured area, swelling, possible deformity, and sometimes bleeding. If you suspect a bone has been broken, the most important thing is to protect the limb from further injury.

Classifications Of Fractures From The American Medical Association

- **Simple:** The bone is broken in one place.
- **Comminuted:** The bone is broken in many places and there are bone fragments present.
- **Open Or Compound:** A compound fracture occurs when the bone protrudes through the skin. Bacteria and other organisms may enter the wound and therefore, the chance of infection is very high.
- **Closed:** The broken bone does not protrude through the skin.
- **Undisplaced:** The broken bone is still aligned.
- **Displaced:** The broken bone is no longer aligned and needs to be re-set.

Action

- Call for emergency help if the victim is not responding, having difficulty breathing, bleeding heavily or in intense pain, or if the area near the break site looks deformed.
- If the wound is not bleeding, apply ice (covered with a cloth) to the injured area to help reduce swelling and inflammation.
- If there is bleeding, apply direct pressure by placing a clean cloth or piece of clothing over the injury for several minutes until the bleeding stops. Add new layers over existing ones if bleeding persists.
- Do not try to move the bone back into normal position. The less movement, the better. Keep the person as quiet as possible and immobilize the joints above and below the affected area.

- Aspirin, ibuprofen, or naproxen sodium will help reduce pain and swelling. Acetaminophen will help the pain, but not the swelling.

- You may want to fashion a splint made of a rigid material. The splint should hold the joint above and below the injury immobile.

> ♣ **It's A Fact!!**
> **Spinal Injuries**
>
> Spinal injuries are particularly dangerous. Never move a victim you believe has a spinal injury unless instructed by emergency medical personnel. Following are signs of spinal injuries:
>
> - Visible head injuries
> - Severe pain in the neck and back
> - Weakness, numbness, or paralysis
> - Lack of control of bodily functions
> - Body is positioned or twisted in an unusual manner
> - Victim is incoherent or unresponsive
>
> Source: "Basic First Aid Guidelines," © Muscogee (Creek) Nation Emergency Management.

Burns

The skin is the largest organ in the body. As living tissue, when it is exposed to heat higher than 120 degrees Fahrenheit, damage occurs to the cells. Each year approximately 2 million people seek medical attention for burns.

Classifications Of Burns

- **First Degree Burns:** First degree burns, though painful, are not serious burns. Only the top layer of the skin is affected. These types of burns cause reddening of the skin and heal quickly.

First Aid Basics

- **Second Degree Burns:** Second degree burns cause damage deeper into the skin and result in blisters. Unless the damage is quite extensive, these burns usually heal without scarring.
- **Third Degree Burns:** Third degree burns destroy all the layers of skin. The area of the burn is white or charred. Bone and muscle tissue may also be exposed if the burn is deep enough. These types of injuries need to be treated by a specialist and require skin grafts to prevent scarring.

Treating Minor Burns

- Cool the burn with cold water.
- Apply a cold-water compress.
- Cover with a sterile gauze bandage.
- If the burn blisters, don't pop the blister. Fluid protects against infection.
- Take an over-the-counter pain reliever to relieve discomfort and swelling.

Treating Major Burns

- If a person's skin or clothing is on fire, make him drop to the ground and roll over and over until the flames are extinguished. You may also use a cotton blanket, towel, or carpet to smother the flames.
- If there is a burn source that can be safely eliminated, such as electrical current, turn it off.
- Ensure that you and the victim are not in further danger.
- Call for emergency assistance.
- Check to see if the victim is breathing and if there is a pulse.
- If there are no open wounds, cool the burn with water, not ice. Use cold cloth compresses on burns to hands, feet, and face.
- Do not apply creams, butter, toothpaste, ointment, antiseptic sprays, or other such products on the burn. These can cause infection.
- Don't remove clothing, even if it's burned, but try to be sure the victim is not near smoke or heat.

Chemical Burns

Burns may be caused by chemicals in the home, at work, or school.

- Remove the chemical that caused the burn, trying not to come in direct with it. If the chemical is a powder, brush it from the skin before using water.

- Call for emergency help:
    - if the victim is unconscious,
    - if the victim is having seizures or difficulty breathing, or
    - if the burn is in eyes, or on hands, feet, face, groin, or over a major joint.

- Remove clothing and jewelry exposed to the spilled chemical.

- Flush the affected area with cool, running water for 15–30 minutes.

- Use moist compresses to help relieve pain.

- Protect the burned area by covering it with a clean cloth.

- If chemicals get into a victim's eyes, flush them immediately with running water for at least 20 minutes. Get medical assistance immediately.

Chest Pains

Characteristics Of A Heart Attack

- Intense, prolonged pain that might feel like pressure or heaviness
- Pain radiating from the left shoulder down the arm or pain in both arms, back, or even the jaw and neck. It may feel like severe indigestion
- Nausea, shortness of breath, and intense sweating
- Weakness, restlessness, and anxiousness
- Loss of consciousness

A variety of things, such as a heart attack, injury to the chest, collapsed lung, blood clot in the lung, anxiety and stress, a pulled muscle, or heartburn can cause chest pain.

First Aid Basics

> ♣ **It's A Fact!!**
> **Electrical Burns**
>
> All electrical burns should be evaluated by a physician. The burn may appear to be minor but may extend deep into the tissue or affect other systems such as the heart.
>
> Source: "Basic First Aid Guidelines," © Muscogee (Creek) Nation Emergency Management.

It is important to take chest pain seriously. Monitor the condition closely, and if you are concerned, see a physician.

It's sometimes difficult to decide whether chest pain is a medical emergency, but the following are highlights of a medical crisis.

Get emergency assistance if the chest pain is accompanied by:

- pain that spreads to the arm, jaw, shoulders, or neck;
- breathing difficulties;
- a feeling of pressure on the left side;
- nausea or vomiting;
- sweating or anxiety; or
- an uneven heartbeat.

These symptoms could indicate the victim is having a heart attack. Heart attacks can cause several minutes of prolonged pain in the chest or can be "silent" with no symptoms.

If you believe someone is experiencing a heart attack, help them sit comfortably and loosen any tight clothing. Get help immediately!

Not Breathing, No Pulse

If a person is not breathing and has no pulse, you need to seek emergency help immediately and be prepared to help the victim until emergency help arrives.

ABCs Of CPR

These are often called the ABCs of CPR—Airway, Breathing, Circulation.

- Open the airway by tilting the head back and lifting the chin.
- Rescue Breathing: perform mouth-to-mouth breathing for the victim.
- Chest Compression: apply systematic pressure at the bottom of the breastbone to maintain blood flow, thus replacing the heartbeat.

Note: Below is a brief description of the steps in CPR. The information is not intended as a substitute for formal CPR training.

Before starting CPR:

- Look at your surroundings to check for safety.
- Tap the victim's shoulder and try to get a response.
- If there is no response, call 911 for emergency assistance, or direct someone else to call.

To perform rescue breathing and chest compressions:

- Tilt the victim's head back. Look, listen and feel for breathing. If the victim isn't breathing normally, pinch closed his nose, cover his mouth with yours, and blow into his mouth twice.
- As you are breathing, watch for the victim's chest to rise.
- If the victim is still not breathing, begin chest compressions. Place your hands in the middle of the victim's chest, directly between his nipples. Push down 30 times. You should compress the chest about two inches.
- After 30 compressions, give the victim two breaths. After four cycles of breaths and compressions, recheck for signs of breathing or circulation. Continue CPR until signs of life return or paramedics arrive to take over.

Seizures And Convulsions

Seizures are episodes of unusual behavior caused by abnormal brain activity. During seizures, victims may cry out, lose consciousness, and jerk and twitch uncontrollably, or they may stare off into space. Most people associate seizures with epilepsy, but other causes include high fevers, low blood sugar, drug overdose, infection, brain injury infections, and any other condition that causes a change in the brain's electrical activity. Most episodes last one to five minutes.

Most seizures stop on their own, but there are a few things you can do to help individuals having seizures:

- Move the victim only if he is in danger or near something hazardous
- Cushion his head with a soft material
- Turn the victim onto his side so he doesn't choke
- Loosen tight clothing around the neck

Do not:

- Place anything in the victim's mouth
- Give medication, food, or water
- Try to restrain his movements

Call for emergency help if the victim has trouble breathing, turns bluish in skin color, has a seizure after suffering a head injury, has diabetes or a heart condition, is pregnant, or may have taken any type of poison or hazardous substances. You should also call 911 if the victim has never had a seizure before or if he doesn't awaken soon after symptoms subside.

Unconsciousness

Loss of consciousness can be caused by major illness, injury, or drug abuse. People can also faint due to low blood sugar, dehydration, temporary low blood pressure, strenuous coughing, hyperventilating, and many other reasons. Some symptoms that may indicate a person is about to lose consciousness include unresponsiveness, light-headedness, disorientation, nausea, drowsiness, and stupor.

If someone begins to "feel faint" he should lean forward and lower his head toward his knees to improve blood flow to the brain.

If someone loses consciousness:

- call for emergency help,
- cushion the victim's head with a soft material,
- look inside the victim's mouth to make sure his airway is unobstructed and check his breathing and pulse,
- open the victim's airway by tilting the head up and lifting the chin, and
- if the victim is not breathing, initiate CPR.

Table 3.1. Basic First Aid Procedures**

<u>Injury</u>	<u>Treatment</u>
Nose Bleeds	Pinch nose and tilt head forward.
Animal Bites	Wash wound, identify animal, and report the bite.
Serious Falls	Do not move the victim; call 9-1-1.
Severe Wounds	Have the victim sit or lie down, apply direct pressure to stop the bleeding, call 9-1-1.
Small Wounds	Wash the wound, apply dressing and bandage.
Bruises	Apply a cold compress.
Burns*	1st and 2nd degree: Put burn in cold water, pat dry, and cover with clean bandage. Do not break blisters.
	3rd degree: Do not put water on an open wound, do not remove burned on clothing. Cover the burn lightly and get medical help!

*A 1st degree burn is red, sore, and covers a small area.
*A 2nd degree burn is blistered and painful.
*A 3rd degree burn causes the skin to be white or charred and there is a loss of skin layers.
**For all severe wounds and burns, dial 911.

Source: Excerpted from an undated document accessed February 18, 2008: "Basic First Aid Procedures," © City of Miami Department of Fire-Rescue (www.ci.miami.fl.us/Fire). Reprinted with permission.

Chapter 4

CPR: Cardiopulmonary Resuscitation

If you've ever watched a hospital show on TV, you've probably seen cardiopulmonary resuscitation (say: kar-dee-o-**pul**-muh-ner-ee rih-suh-sih-**tay**-shun). That's when a doctor or another rescuer breathes into someone's mouth and presses on the person's chest. It's called CPR for short and it saves lives. Let's find out how it works.

What is CPR?

Cardio means "of the heart" and pulmonary means "of the lungs." Resuscitation is a medical word that means "to revive"—or bring back to life. Sometimes CPR can help a person who has stopped breathing, and whose heart may have stopped beating, to stay alive.

People who handle emergencies—such as police officers, firefighters, paramedics, doctors, and nurses—are all trained to do CPR. Many other teens and adults—like lifeguards, teachers, child-care workers, and maybe even your mom or dad—know how to do CPR as well.

Here's what takes place during CPR: A person giving CPR—called a rescuer—will give some breaths to someone who is not breathing on his or her

---

About This Chapter: "CPR: A Real Lifesaver," August 2006, reprinted with permission from www.kidshealth.org. Copyright © 2006 The Nemours Foundation. This information was provided by KidsHealth, one of the largest resources online for medically reviewed health information written for parents, kids, and teens. For more articles like this one, visit www.KidsHealth.org, or www.TeensHealth.org.

own. This is called artificial respiration (say: ar-tuh-**fih**-shul res-puh-**ray**-shun), mouth-to-mouth rescue breathing, or mouth-to-mouth resuscitation.

To do this, a rescuer puts his or her mouth over the other person's open mouth and blows, forcing air into the lungs. (Ideally the rescuer will use a special mask so that their mouths don't actually have to touch.) Rescue breathing helps to move oxygen, which everyone needs to live, down into the lungs of the person who isn't breathing.

After giving two breaths, the rescuer will probably use both hands, one placed over the other, to press on the person's chest many times in a row to move blood out of a heart that has stopped beating. These are called chest compressions and they help move oxygen-carrying blood to the body's vital organs—especially the all-important brain. A person who goes too long without oxygen reaching the brain will die. After 30 chest compressions have been given, two more rescue breaths are given and the cycle continues until help arrives.

In between chest compressions, the person's rib cage relaxes long enough to let blood flow back toward the heart. In this way, the rescuer can keep the person alive by continuing to supply blood and oxygen to the brain and the rest of the body, until emergency help—like the paramedics—arrives to take the person to a hospital.

Instead of doing mouth-to-mouth rescue breathing, professional rescuers—such as paramedics—will provide artificial breathing for someone by using a mask with a special hand pump connected to an oxygen tank. Doctors in the emergency department will put a tube into the person's windpipe to pump oxygen directly through the tube and into the lungs.

When should someone use CPR?

The steps in CPR should be used whenever someone is not breathing and when the heart is not beating. After a couple of rescue breaths are given, 30 chest compressions should be started right away.

Someone can stop breathing or have cardiac arrest from:
- heart attacks;
- strokes (when the blood flow to a part of the brain suddenly stops);

CPR: Cardiopulmonary Resuscitation

- choking on something that blocks the entire airway;
- near-drowning incidents (when someone is under water for too long and stops breathing);
- a very bad neck, head, or back injury;
- severe electrical shocks (like from touching a power line);
- being very sick from a serious infection;
- too much bleeding; or
- severe allergic reactions.

Who should know CPR?

Certain people need to know how to perform CPR to do their jobs. Medical professionals—from nurses and doctors to paramedics and emergency medicine technicians—must know CPR. Lifeguards, child-care workers, school coaches, and trainers usually have to learn CPR. Many parents know how to perform CPR on their children in case of emergency. Other adults who have family members with medical conditions such as heart disease sometimes know CPR, too.

> ✔ **Quick Tip**
>
> If an emergency happens or someone becomes very sick while you're around, do your best to stay calm. First, try to get the person to respond by gently shaking his or her shoulder and asking, "Are you OK?" If there is no response and you are certified in CPR, you can begin CPR. If you're alone, shout for help or call 911 yourself.

Many people—maybe you—may want to learn how to do CPR just in case they need to use it someday. You can never tell when a medical emergency will happen and it feels good to know that you could help. The American Red Cross, American Heart Association, and the National Safety Council all offer CPR courses. You also might find CPR classes at your local hospital, places of worship, the YMCA, or your school. You are usually ready to take a CPR course and get certified if you are in middle school or above.

Talk with your mom or dad if you'd like to learn how to do it. Knowing CPR can be a real lifesaver!

Chapter 5

Emergency Department Visits

Millions of Americans visit an emergency room each year. Millions more have seen the hit TV show *ER*. This has sparked an almost insatiable interest in the fascinating, 24-hour-a-day, non-stop world of emergency medicine. A visit to the emergency room can be a stressful, scary event. Why is it so scary? First of all, there is the fear of not knowing what is wrong with you. There is the fear of having to visit an unfamiliar place filled with people you have never met. Also, you may have to undergo tests that you do not understand at a pace that discourages questions and comprehension.

This chapter leads you through a complete behind-the-scenes tour of a typical emergency room. You will learn about the normal flow of traffic in an emergency room, the people involved, and the special techniques used to respond to life-or-death situations. If you yourself find the need to visit an emergency room, this information will make it less stressful by revealing what will happen and why things happen the way they do in an emergency department.

Emergency Room Patients

One of the most amazing aspects of emergency medicine is the huge range of conditions that arrive on a daily basis. No other specialty in medicine sees the variety of conditions that an emergency room physician sees in

---

About This Chapter: Text in this chapter is from "How Emergency Rooms Work," by Carl Bianco, M.D., © 2008. Reprinted courtesy of HowStuffWorks.com.

a typical week. Some of the conditions that bring people to the emergency room include:

- Car accidents;
- Sports injuries;
- Broken bones and cuts from accidents and falls;
- Burns;
- Uncontrolled bleeding;
- Heart attacks, chest pain;
- Difficulty breathing, asthma attacks, pneumonia;
- Strokes, loss of function and/or numbness in arms or legs;
- Loss of vision, hearing;
- Unconsciousness;
- Confusion, altered level of consciousness, fainting;
- Suicidal or homicidal thoughts;
- Overdoses;
- Severe abdominal pain, persistent vomiting;
- Food poisoning;
- Blood when vomiting, coughing, urinating, or in bowel movements;
- Severe allergic reactions from insect bites, foods, or medications;
- Complications from diseases, high fevers.

Understanding The ER Maze

The classic emergency room scene involves an ambulance screeching to a halt, a gurney hurtling through the hallway and five people frantically working to save a person's life with only seconds to spare. This does happen and is not uncommon, but the majority of cases seen in a typical emergency department aren't quite this dramatic. Let's look at a typical case to see how the normal flow of an emergency room works.

Emergency Department Visits

Imagine that it's 2 a.m., and you're dreaming about whatever it is that you dream about. Suddenly you wake up because your abdomen hurts—a lot. This seems like something out of the ordinary, so you call your regular doctor. He tells you to go to your local hospital's emergency department: He is concerned about appendicitis because your pain is located in the right, lower abdomen.

Triage

When you arrive at the Emergency Department, your first stop is triage. This is the place where each patient's condition is prioritized, typically by a nurse, into three general categories. The categories are:

- immediately life threatening;
- urgent, but not immediately life threatening; and
- less urgent.

This categorization is necessary so that someone with a life-threatening condition is not kept waiting because they arrive a few minutes later than someone with a more routine problem. The triage nurse records your vital signs (temperature, pulse, respiratory rate, and blood pressure). She also gets a brief history of your current medical complaints, past medical problems, medications, and allergies so that she can determine the appropriate triage category. Here you find out that your temperature is 101 degrees F.

What's next? You need to register.

Registration

After triage, the next stop is registration—not very exciting and rarely seen on TV. Here they obtain your vital statistics. You may also provide them with your insurance information, Medicare, Medicaid, or HMO card. This step is necessary to develop a medical record so that your medical history, lab tests, x-rays, etc., will all be located on one chart that can be referenced at any time. The bill will also be generated from this information.

If the patient's condition is life-threatening or if the patient arrives by ambulance, this step may be completed later at the bedside.

Examination Room

Now you are brought to the exam room. You promptly throw up in the bathroom, which may be more evidence of appendicitis. You are seen by an emergency-department nurse who obtains more detailed information about you. The nurse gets you settled into a patient gown so that you can be examined properly and perhaps obtains a urine specimen at this time.

♣ **It's A Fact!!**
About Money: All patients must receive a medical screening exam regardless of their ability to pay.

Some emergency departments have been subdivided into separate areas to better serve their patients. These separate areas can include a pediatric ER, a chest-pain ER, a fast track (for minor injuries and illnesses), trauma center (usually for severely injured patients), and an observation unit (for patients who do not require hospital admission but do require prolonged treatment or many diagnostic tests).

Once the nurse has finished her tasks, the next visitor is an emergency-medicine physician. He gets a more detailed medical history about your present illness, past medical problems, family history, social history, and a complete review of all your body systems. He then formulates a list of possible causes of your symptoms. This list is called a differential diagnosis. The most likely diagnosis is then determined by the patient's symptoms and physical examination. If this is inadequate to determine the diagnosis, then diagnostic tests are required.

Who's On First

The vast array of people caring for patients in an emergency department can be quite confusing to the average health care consumer—as confusing as if you were watching your first baseball game ever and no one was around to explain all those players.

Additionally, most people are uncertain of the training and background necessary to become a member of the emergency-department team. Well, here's the scorecard.

Emergency Physician

The emergency physician comes to the team after spending four years in college studying hard to get as high a GPA (grade point average) as possible in order to get accepted into medical school.

Medical school is a four-year course of study covering all the essentials of becoming a physician. It generally includes two years of classroom time, followed by two years rotating through all the different specialties of medicine.

Toward the end of medical school, each medical student must select a particular specialty (emergency medicine, family practice, internal medicine, surgery, pediatrics, etc.). The medical student then completes an internship (one year) and residency (two to three additional years) in order to be a specialist in emergency medicine.

Physicians must pass an all-day written exam and an all-day oral exam to become board certified in emergency medicine. As of 2001, there were approximately 32,000 emergency physicians practicing in the United States, of which 17,000 were certified by the American Board of Emergency Medicine.

Emergency Nurse

The emergency nurse comes to the team in a number of ways. One way is completing a four-year degree in college to obtain a BSN. (bachelor of science in nursing). Alternately, a nurse may complete a three-year diploma program (usually at a hospital) or a two-year associates degree program (usually at a community college). After completing any of these academic endeavors, the nursing graduate is eligible to take a licensing exam. After passing this exam, the nursing graduate becomes an RN (registered nurse) and can practice nursing. Many emergency nurses take an additional exam to become a CEN (Certified Emergency Nurse).

Physician Assistant

Many emergency departments utilize physician assistants (PA). PAs work under the supervision of an emergency physician. They can examine, diagnose, and treat patients (usually the less complicated ones) and review their findings with the physician. In most states, they can prescribe medications.

Typically, a PA has at least two years of college (most have a four-year degree) and some health-care experience before completing a two-year program to become a physician assistant. An exam is required to become licensed.

Emergency Department Technician

Many emergency departments have emergency technicians who perform a variety of tasks depending on the institution and state laws. Some of these tasks may include taking your vital signs, drawing your blood, starting your IV, performing EKGs, transporting you to and from various tests, and providing aid and comfort to family and friends. Training varies widely, but these technicians are often ambulance personnel or else are trained through the hospital.

Unit Secretary

This essential member of the team is one you don't hear about very often. He/she often handles the communication needs of the ER. A few important examples of important communication needs include the emergency physician needing to speak to the patient's family physician, families calling about their loved ones, family physicians needing to inform the emergency department about patients being sent in, or patients calling in needing medical advice. Also, he/she coordinates the ordering of diagnostic tests.

Disposition

Depending on a patient's specific medical condition, physicians will either admit the patient to the hospital, discharge the patient, or transfer the patient to a more appropriate medical facility.

If you are discharged, you will receive discharge instructions (either written specifically for you or pre-printed) that explain your medications and other treatments. If medications are prescribed, you may receive a beginning dose if there are no pharmacies open in your area at that particular time. You will also be referred for follow-up care should your condition continue or worsen.

You may need to be transferred if your condition is better treated at another institution. You may have to sign a consent form if your condition or mental state allows.

The modern emergency department performs an important role in our society. It really is a marvelous invention that has saved countless lives. Hopefully, the information in this chapter will help ease your fears should you need the services of an emergency department in the future.

♣ It's A Fact!!

Physicians In Training

At teaching hospitals, you may be examined by an intern or resident. Teaching hospitals are hospitals that have training programs for physicians and are usually affiliated with a medical school. Interns are in their first year of training after graduating medical school. After the first year, the physician in training is called a resident. These physicians are supervised by an attending physician who usually has extensive experience in emergency medicine.

Chapter 6

Hospitalization

You might go to the hospital if you fall off your bike and break your arm or if you have asthma and have trouble breathing. You might go to the hospital if you become dehydrated and need IV fluids or if you need to have surgery to take out your tonsils.

It may seem a little scary to go to a hospital, but doctors, nurses, and other hospital workers are there to help people who are sick or hurt feel better. Read on to find out what happens inside a hospital.

Admissions

Sometimes, your doctor decides you need to be admitted to the hospital (that means you will stay overnight). He or she either needs to find out about something going on inside your body or has decided you need special medicine, surgery, or other treatment for a health problem. Your doctor will call the hospital to tell the staff that you're coming, and you will go to the admissions office to check in.

Another way that kids are admitted to the hospital is through the emergency room. You might go to the emergency room if you are very sick,

> About This Chapter: " Going to the Hospital," April 2007, reprinted with permission from www.kidshealth.org. Copyright © 2007 The Nemours Foundation. This information was provided by KidsHealth, one of the largest resources online for medically reviewed health information written for parents, kids, and teens. For more articles like this one, visit www.KidsHealth.org, or www.TeensHealth.org.

especially if your doctor or parent feels that you need medical attention right away. In the emergency room, the doctors and nurses will take care of you and help you feel better. If you need to stay overnight at the hospital, someone from the hospital staff will take you and your parents to your hospital room.

When you go into the hospital, you will probably see your mom or dad fill out a lot of different papers. It's important that the hospital has your name, address, phone number, birth date, and other information, like if you take any medicines or have any allergies. You might be asked a lot of questions (sometimes again and again) like your name, your birthday, and how you are feeling. If you don't understand a question, it can help to ask your parents—or the doctor or nurse taking care of you—to explain.

Your Room

Once you're in the hospital, you may have a room all to yourself or sometimes you will share one with another child. Your room will have a bed, usually with buttons to push that will make the bed move up or down. A curtain can be pulled around your bed so that you can have some privacy while you're resting or changing clothes. There are usually lights that you can turn on and off, and there is a special button to push that will call the nurse if you need anything. You'll probably have a bathroom in your room.

Many hospital rooms have a TV and a telephone to help you keep busy while you're in the hospital. If you're going to be in the hospital for a little while, you can always bring things that remind you of home, like pictures of your family, stuffed animals, books, or toys—or even put up favorite pictures or posters on the wall around your bed. You may want to bring your favorite pillow and blanket to be more comfortable.

Your Clothes

In many hospitals, you can wear anything you want—like your own pajamas or bathrobe. Sometimes you might have to wear a special hospital gown that makes it easier for the doctor or nurse to examine you. The hospital usually provides slipper socks or you can bring your own.

Hospital People

You'll meet lots of people in the hospital, from the moment you arrive until you're ready to leave. You might meet as many as 30 people just on your first day.

You'll meet nurses who will help admit you to the hospital and show you around the hospital floor so you'll know where things are. While you're in the hospital, nurses will take care of you day and night. They'll check on you throughout the day to see how you're feeling and if you need anything to be comfortable. Every few hours, they'll take your temperature and blood pressure and listen to your heart and lungs. Nurses will also bring you any medicines you may need while you're sick.

You'll see plenty of doctors in the hospital, too. You might see your own doctor or a doctor who always works in the hospital and takes care of children. If you're in a hospital just for kids, you'll probably also see medical students (who are learning to be doctors) and residents (doctors receiving special training in taking care of kids).

You also might see a medical specialist—that's a doctor who is an expert in a certain kind of medical problem or part of the body. A cardiologist—a doctor who specializes in taking care of the heart—is one example of a specialist.

Another example is if you have asthma and need to be in the hospital, you might see a lung specialist or allergist who will help you with your breathing problems.

Transport people will take you from place to place; volunteers may bring coffee to parents or play games and watch videos with kids in the playroom; and therapists will show you how to use pieces of equipment, like crutches, if you need them.

> ♣ **It's A Fact!!**
> **Your Family**
>
> Almost every hospital will let one of your parents stay with you all the time, even while you're sleeping in your room. During the day, sisters, brothers, grandparents, and friends can visit. They might even bring you flowers, balloons, or other treats.

Some hospitals have child life specialists. A child life specialist's job is to make sure kids in the hospital understand what's going on around them and help them feel more comfortable. Child life specialists can help explain something a doctor or nurse will do, like place an IV or take someone to the operating room for surgery. They can make these things seem less scary.

Getting Tests

You will probably have some tests while you're in the hospital—not the kind you take in school! The doctor may order a blood test, which involves taking some blood from a vein in your arm. This test can pinch a little, but it won't hurt too much. For other kinds of tests, you may need to give some urine (pee).

Sometimes an x-ray, computed tomography (CT) scan, or magnetic resonance imaging (MRI) will need to be done. These tests use a special camera to take a picture of a part of your body. This helps doctors see the bones and tissues inside your body and helps them to see if anything is wrong or is making you sick. If there is a test you don't understand, you can ask the doctor or nurse about it, and they will explain it to you.

Having Surgery

If you have surgery (that's another name for having an operation), you will meet an anesthesiologist (say: an-us-**thee**-zee-al-uh-jist) before the operation. The job of an anesthesiologist is to help you sleep during the surgery with special medicines. This way you won't feel anything while your doctor operates on you.

On the day of surgery, you won't be able to eat breakfast because you can't have an operation on a full stomach. But don't worry—your body will get fluids through an IV. An IV is a tiny tube that carries medicine or fluids into your body through a vein, usually in your arm or hand.

When it's time for the operation, a transport person will wheel you on a special bed to the operating room, where you'll get anesthesia to go to sleep. While you're still awake, the hospital staff will explain everything that is going to happen. If you have any questions, you should always ask.

After your operation, when you wake up, you'll either be back in your room or in a special recovery room—that's a room where nurses can keep checking on you to make sure you're OK.

Keeping Busy

Most hospitals have playrooms, where you'll find toys, arts and crafts, and games. Someone will be there to help you find something to do. If you can't go to the playroom, someone can bring you things to play with. Most hospitals have TVs or video games, and many have computers (with games) that can be brought to your bed. Also, many hospitals have special visitors stop by, like clowns or story characters.

Keeping Up With Schoolwork

If you're worried about falling behind on schoolwork while you're in the hospital, there are ways to keep up. Many children's hospitals have a classroom and a teacher for kids who are in the hospital for a while. For shorter stays, if you feel up to it, your parents can have your schoolwork sent home or to the hospital. If you're not feeling great and you don't think you can keep up with the schoolwork, your school will understand and give you extra time when you go back.

Being Nervous ♣ It's A Fact!!

It's normal to be a little nervous—and even scared—when going to the hospital. But remember:

- Your family will be with you.

- There are other kids in the hospital who are going through the same kind of thing.

- Lots of people, like doctors and nurses, can answer any questions you might have. Don't be afraid to ask. Remember, they're there to help you feel better and will be glad to make you more comfortable.

- After spending time at the hospital, you should be on the road to feeling better.

Chapter 7

Coping With A Traumatic Experience

Questions And Answers About Traumatic Events

What is a traumatic event?

Most everyone has been through a stressful event in his or her life. When the event, or series of events, causes a lot of stress, it is called a traumatic event. Traumatic events are marked by a sense of horror, helplessness, serious injury, or the threat of serious injury or death. Traumatic events affect survivors, rescue workers, and the friends and relatives of victims who have been involved. They may also have an impact on people who have seen the event either firsthand or on television.

What are some common responses?

A person's response to a traumatic event may vary. Responses include feelings of fear, grief, and depression. Physical and behavioral responses include nausea, dizziness, and changes in appetite and sleep pattern as well as withdrawal from daily activities. Responses to trauma can last for weeks to months before people start to feel normal again.

About This Chapter: This chapter begins with excerpts from "Coping with a Traumatic Event," Centers for Disease Control and Prevention (CDC), July 26, 2005. Additional information is from "School Violence: Tips for Coping with Stress," CDC, February 14, 2008.

Most people report feeling better within three months after a traumatic event. If the problems become worse or last longer than one month after the event, the person may be suffering from post-traumatic stress disorder (PTSD).

What is PTSD?

Post-traumatic stress disorder (PTSD) is an intense physical and emotional response to thoughts and reminders of the event that last for many weeks or months after the traumatic event. The symptoms of PTSD fall into three broad types: re-living, avoidance, and increased arousal.

- Symptoms of re-living include flashbacks, nightmares, and extreme emotional and physical reactions to reminders of the event. Emotional reactions can include feeling guilty, extreme fear of harm, and numbing of emotions. Physical reactions can include uncontrollable shaking, chills or heart palpitations, and tension headaches.

- Symptoms of avoidance include staying away from activities, places, thoughts, or feelings related to the trauma or feeling detached or estranged from others.

- Symptoms of increased arousal include being overly alert or easily startled, difficulty sleeping, irritability or outbursts of anger, and lack of concentration.

Other symptoms linked with PTSD include: panic attacks, depression, suicidal thought and feelings, drug abuse, feelings of being estranged and isolated, and not being able to complete daily tasks.

What can you do for yourself?

There are many things you can do to cope with traumatic events.

- Understand that your symptoms may be normal, especially right after the trauma.
- Keep to your usual routine.
- Take the time to resolve day-to-day conflicts so they do not add to your stress.

- Do not shy away from situations, people and places that remind you of the trauma.
- Find ways to relax and be kind to yourself.
- Turn to family, friends, and clergy person for support, and talk about your experiences and feelings with them.
- Participate in leisure and recreational activities.
- Recognize that you cannot control everything.
- Recognize the need for trained help, and call a local mental health center.

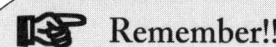

Remember!!

Remember that it is all right to:

- feel upset when something bad or scary happens.
- express feelings and thoughts, without making judgments.
- return to daily routines.

Source: CDC, 2005.

When should you contact your doctor or mental health professional?

About half of those with PTSD recover within three months without treatment. Sometimes symptoms do not go away on their own or they last for more than three months. This may happen because of the severity of the event, direct exposure to the traumatic event, seriousness of the threat to life, the number of times an event happened, a history of past trauma, and psychological problems before the event.

You may need to consider seeking professional help if your symptoms affect your relationship with your family and friends, or affect your job. If you suspect that you or someone you know has PTSD, talk with a health care provider or call your local mental health clinic.

School Violence: Tips For Coping

Common Reactions To Tragedies Vary

Tragedies, including school shootings, affect different people in different ways. Understanding how this traumatic event may affect you can be useful as you begin to get back to your typical routines and relationships. Keep in mind that returning to your normal routine can take some time.

You may have witnessed the loss of life, experienced feelings of grief, sadness, and suffering, experienced separation or lack of communication with family, friends and co-workers. At some point you may have felt that your own health and safety or the health and safety of someone you care about was in danger.

It is common for people who experience a tragedy to:

- feel a sense of loss, sadness, frustration, helplessness, or emotional numbness,
- experience troubling memories from that day,
- have nightmares or difficulty falling or staying asleep,
- have no desire for food or a loss of appetite,
- have difficulty concentrating, or
- feel nervous or on edge.

Some people may notice positive changes as a result of this situation, such as increased respect for life and personal relationships.

Talk about your experiences and get support from your family, friends, and co-workers. Other places to seek support can include faith-based or volunteer organizations, such as the local American Red Cross.

It is important to take care of yourself by keeping your normal routine. Avoid using alcohol and drugs which can suppress your feelings rather than letting them come out. Helping other people or volunteering in your community can help you feel better as well. Keep in mind that returning to the way you felt before the event may take some time.

Tips For Students

Whether or not you were directly affected by a violent event, it is normal to feel anxious about your own safety and to want to make sense of the situation. The Centers for Disease Control (CDC) offers these suggestions to help kids and teens cope with the aftermath of a traumatic event.

Coping With A Traumatic Experience

> ✔ **Quick Tip**
>
> If you or someone you know needs immediate help please contact the one of the following crisis hotlines:
>
> - Youth Crisis Number: 800-499-9130
> - Youth Mental Health Line: 888-568-1112
> - Child-Help USA: 800-422-4453 (24 hour toll free)
> - National Suicide Prevention Lifeline: 800-273-TALK (888-628-9454 for Spanish-speaking callers)
>
> Source: CDC, 2008.

Talk to an adult you trust: This might be your parent, another relative, a friend, neighbor, teacher, coach, school nurse, guidance counselor, member of the clergy, or family doctor. If you've witnessed or experienced violence of any kind, not talking about it can make feelings build up inside and cause problems. If you are not sure where to turn, call your local crisis intervention center or a national hotline.

Stay active: Go for a walk, volunteer with a community group, play sports, write a play or poem, play a musical instrument, or join a club or after-school program. Trying any of these can be a positive way to handle your emotions.

Take the initiative to make your school or community safer: Join an existing group that is promoting non-violence in your school or community, or launch your own effort. Safeyouth.org (www.safeyouth.org) can connect you with national organizations and provide you with information and resources to take action in your community.

Stay in touch with family: If possible, stay in touch with trusted family, friends, and neighbors to talk things out and help deal with any stress or worry.

Part Two
Medical Emergencies And Traumatic Injuries

Chapter 8

Bites And Stings

Bug Bites And Stings

Bug bites and stings are, for the most part, no more unpleasant than a homework assignment—kind of annoying but basically harmless. Occasionally, though, an insect bite or sting can cause serious problems. You should know when a simple ice pack can bring some relief or when a visit to the local hospital is in order.

Know Your Enemy

Before you find out how to handle your unwelcome guests, come meet the critters who want a little piece of you.

The Biters: Mosquitoes hang out anywhere people, food, or pools of still water are found. Generally they aren't anything to worry about: They bite, you itch, end of story.

However, there is some concern about West Nile virus, which is transmitted to humans by mosquitoes. The good news is that healthy kids, teens,

---

About This Chapter: This chapter begins with "Bug Bites and Stings," September 2007, reprinted with permission from www.kidshealth.org. Copyright © 2007 The Nemours Foundation. This information was provided by KidsHealth, one of the largest resources online for medically reviewed health information written for parents, kids, and teens. For more articles like this one, visit www.KidsHealth.org, or www.TeensHealth.org. Additional information from the American Academy of Family Physicians is cited separately within the chapter.

and adults under 50 are at low risk of catching West Nile virus. And although the virus can put people at risk for developing a serious infection called encephalitis, in reality this hardly ever happens. Less than 1% of the people who are infected with West Nile virus become seriously ill.

Fleas can be lumped into the irritating-but-not-serious category as well. They are often found on Fido or Fluffy, but they can also be attracted to you.

Depending on where you live, ticks could ruin a good camping trip. One variety known as deer ticks is known to carry Lyme disease, so the trick is to get them off your body fast. In the United States, the northeastern and upper midwestern states are most affected by the threat of disease from ticks, but some cases have been found in the Pacific Northwest and in northern and southern Europe. Ticks can carry other diseases, too, such as Rocky Mountain spotted fever. Ticks are usually found in heavily wooded areas.

Most spider bites are minor, although they can cause mild swelling or allergic reactions. But a small percentage of teens become ill after being bitten by brown recluse or black widow spiders. Although not everyone will have a reaction, you should see a doctor and get treatment quickly if you know you've been bitten by one of these spiders.

The brown recluse is brown (big surprise) with a small shape of a violin in a darker brown area on the back of its head. These spiders are small but tough: a half-inch body (about one centimeter) with legs stretching another inch (three centimeters) or even more. They are found mostly in the southern central part of the United States, and they like to hide in dark, quiet places like attics or garages. When humans enter their space unexpectedly, they bite out of fear. The bites usually don't hurt at first—and most people don't even know that they've been bitten.

Brown recluse bites don't cause problems for most people. But in a small percentage of cases, they can lead to skin damage and scarring. The few people who do have a reaction may notice swelling and skin changes four to eight hours after the bite. The swelling may form a blister. If this happens, a dark, scabby material called eschar (pronounced: **es**-kar) may cover the blister within a week after the bite. Most brown recluse bites get better on their own—but it can take a couple of months. So it's always a good idea to see a doctor for proper treatment.

The black widow is found in southern Canada, throughout the United States, and in Mexico. Easily identified by its shiny coal-black body and orange hourglass shape on its underbelly, it's a similar size to the brown recluse spider and it should be treated as carefully.

Most often, people who have been bitten by a black widow don't even know it until they feel the symptoms. But the good news is that there are lots of warning signs that give you time to act before things get too serious. The venom (poison) in a black widow bite causes what's called a systemic reaction, meaning that the poison causes a reaction throughout a person's body, not just around the bite area.

Someone who has been bitten by a black widow may get painful cramps within a few hours. These cramps usually make a person feel achy all over, and can spread to include abdominal cramping, which may be severe. The person may also have nausea, vomiting, chills, fever, and headache. If you show any of these symptoms, get to the hospital immediately.

The Stingers: For most people, being stung by a bee is a minor nuisance. The affected area may get a little red or swollen and it may be slightly painful, but that's about it.

Bees and wasps carry a sting that can cause real problems for people who are allergic, though. As with spider bites, a person can get a localized allergic reaction (swelling, heat, or itching of the skin around the bite area) or a systemic allergic reaction.

In the case of a systemic reaction, the person may break out in hives. Other symptoms include wheezing; shortness of breath; rapid heartbeat; faintness; and swelling of the face, lips,

♣ **It's A Fact!!**
Spider bites can sound scary, but it's actually extremely rare that a person will die from one. Fewer than 1% of the people who report being bitten by a black widow die, and even fewer people die from brown recluse bites. Young children are most at risk.

Source: Nemours Foundation, September 2007.

or tongue. If a person has these symptoms, it's important to get help immediately. It hardly ever happens, but severe allergic reactions to bee stings can be fatal if the person doesn't get medical help.

Once Bitten, Twice Sly

For most varieties of bug bites and stings, antihistamines will help to stop itching and lessen swelling, and acetaminophen can help relieve any pain. Ibuprofen can help reduce swelling while relieving some pain. Some people use a topical steroid cream like hydrocortisone to alleviate itching.

Say goodbye to ticks by removing them with a pair of tweezers as soon as you notice them. Ticks removed within 24 to 48 hours are less likely to transmit diseases like Lyme disease. Be sure to pull a tick out from the head, which is closest to your skin, to ensure that you remove the whole thing. Have someone help you get the hard-to-reach places of your body, and pull each one out very slowly. Clean the site with soap and water, and treat with an antiseptic or antibiotic cream to avoid infection.

Do not try to burn a tick off, as the flame only agitates the insect, causing it to burrow deeper into your skin. When you've pulled the tick out, put it in a jar of rubbing alcohol to kill it. (Your doctor may also want you to save the tick so that its type can be identified.)

After a bee sting, if you can see the stinger, remove it as quickly as possible to lessen your exposure to the venom.

Wash the sting or bite with soap and water and keep it clean. Apply some calamine lotion or a paste of water and baking soda (unless the sting is near your eyes). Put an ice pack on the affected area for 15 minutes every few hours or so, or cover the sting with a cold compress. Apply an antibiotic cream to prevent further infection. Using a 1% hydrocortisone cream (sold in pharmacies without a prescription) can reduce redness, swelling, itching, and pain.

If you are allergic to bee stings, see your doctor for a prescription for an epinephrine kit. If used immediately after a bee attack, this shot will stop the allergic reaction before it starts, which could save your life. An epinephrine kit is easy to use—your doctor or pharmacist will explain how.

Bites And Stings

If you're severely allergic to bug bites and stings, talk to a doctor about getting venom immunotherapy (shots) from an allergist.

Serious Stuff—Seek Medical Help

How do you know when a sting or bite is too much for you to handle alone? If you have any symptoms of a systemic allergic reaction, get to the emergency department right away. These symptoms include:

- shortness of breath;
- wheezing;
- redness or hives over most of your body;
- swelling of the face, lips, or tongue;
- feeling like your throat is closing up;
- nausea;
- vomiting;
- chills;
- muscle aches or cramps;
- weakness;
- fever.

If bites or stings get infected or if an open sore or blister refuses to heal, make an appointment with your family doctor.

> ✔ **Quick Tip**
>
> In the case of a black widow spider bite, or if you have any doubt about what kind of spider bit you and you're feeling sick and have cramps, get to the emergency department immediately. (Take the spider with you if you were able to kill it safely.)
>
> Source: Nemours Foundation, September 2007.

Coulda, Shoulda, Woulda

Human beings don't have to sit around and wait to be a sample on the insect buffet. Here are some steps we can take to protect ourselves:

- Prevent flea infestations by treating your house (including all carpets, furniture, and pets) regularly during the warmer months. Frequent vacuuming can also help.

- Avoid mosquitoes by staying away from areas where mosquitoes breed, such as still pools or ponds, during hot weather. Remove standing water from birdbaths, buckets, etc.; try to stay inside when mosquitoes are most active (dawn and dusk); and wear insect repellent when you are outside.

- When in tick country, take turns with friends and family checking one another for ticks every few hours. Remove any you find immediately. The most important places to check are behind your ears, on your scalp, on the back of your neck, in your armpits, in your groin area, and behind your knees. If you have a pet with you, check your pet, too! Use tick products on pets to prevent them from being bitten.

- Use insect repellent when spending time outdoors camping, hiking, or on the beach. Repellents that contain 10% to 30% DEET (N,N-diethyl-metatoluamide) are approved for mosquitoes, ticks, and some other bugs. Repellents that contain picaridin (KBR 3023) or oil of lemon eucalyptus (p-menthane 3, 8-diol or PMD) are effective against mosquitoes. Follow the instructions carefully and don't overuse the product—using more than you need won't give you any extra protection. Reapply insect repellent after swimming or if you've been sweating for a long time.

- When you are in wooded areas, tuck your clothes in and try to keep as covered up as possible. Tuck pants into socks, shirts into pants, and sleeves into gloves. Wear shoes and socks when walking on grass, even it's just for a minute. Bees and wasps can sting your unprotected feet.

- Wear gloves if you're gardening.

- Don't disturb bee or wasp nests.

- Don't swat at buzzing insects—they will sting if they feel threatened.

- Be aware that spiders might be hiding in undisturbed piles of wood, seldom-opened boxes, or corners behind furniture, and proceed with caution.

Cat And Dog Bites

Reprinted with permission from "Cat and Dog Bites," September 2000, updated June 2008, http://familydoctor.org/online/famdocen/home/healthy/firstaid/bites/203.html. Copyright © 2008 American Academy of Family Physicians. All Rights Reserved.

Bites And Stings

How should I take care of a bite from a cat or a dog?

Here are some things you should do to take care of a wound caused by a cat or dog bite:

- If necessary, call your doctor.
- Wash the wound gently with soap and water.
- Apply pressure with a clean towel to the injured part to stop the bleeding.
- Apply a sterile bandage to the wound.
- Keep the injury elevated above the level of the heart to slow swelling and prevent infection.
- Report the incident to the proper authority in your community (for example, animal control office or police).
- Apply antibiotic ointment to the area two times every day until it heals.

Call your doctor in any of these situations.

- You have a cat bite. Cat bites often cause infection. You don't need to call your doctor for a cat scratch, unless you think the wound is infected.
- You have a dog bite on your hand, foot, or head, or you have a bite that is deep or gaping.
- You have diabetes, liver or lung disease, cancer, acquired immunodeficiency syndrome (AIDS), or another condition that could weaken your ability to fight infection.
- You have any signs of infection, such as redness, swelling, warmth, increased tenderness, oozing of pus from the wound, or fever.
- You have bleeding that doesn't stop after 15 minutes of pressure or you think you may have a broken bone, nerve damage, or another serious injury.
- Your last tetanus shot (vaccine) was more than five years ago. (If so, you may need a booster shot.)

What will my doctor do?

Here are some things your doctor may do to treat a cat or dog bite:

- Examine the wound for possible nerve or tendon damage, or bone injury. He or she will also check for signs of infection.
- Clean the wound with a special solution and remove any damaged tissue.
- May use stitches to close a bite wound, but often the wound is left open to heal, so the risk of infection is lowered.
- May prescribe an antibiotic to prevent infection.
- May give you a tetanus shot if you had your last shot more than five years ago.
- May ask you to schedule an office visit to check your wound again in one to two days.
- If your injury is severe, or if the infection has not gotten better even though you're taking antibiotics, your doctor may suggest that you see a specialist and/or go to the hospital, where you can get special medicine given directly in your veins (intravenous antibiotics) and further treatment if necessary.

Will I need a rabies shot?

Probably not. Rabies is uncommon in dogs and cats in the United States. If a dog or cat that bit you appeared to be healthy at the time of the bite, it's unlikely that the animal had rabies. However, it's a good idea to take some precautions if you're bitten by a dog or cat.

> ✔ Quick Tip
> **How can I prevent cat and dog bites?**
>
> Here are some things you can do to prevent bites:
>
> - Never leave a young child alone with a pet.
> - Do not try to separate fighting animals.
> - Avoid sick animals and animals that you don't know.
> - Leave animals alone while they're eating.
> - Keep pets on a leash when in public.
> - Select your family pet carefully, and be sure to keep your pet's vaccinations (shots) up-to-date.
>
> Source: American Academy of Family Physicians, © 2008.

If you know the owner of the dog or cat that bit you, ask for the pet's vaccination record (record of shots). An animal that appears healthy and has been vaccinated should still be quarantined (kept away from people and other animals) for 10 days to make sure it doesn't start showing signs of rabies. If the animal gets sick during the 10-day period, a veterinarian will test it for rabies. If the animal does have rabies, you will need to get a series of rabies shots.

If the animal is a stray, or you can't find the owner of the dog or cat that bit you, call the animal control agency or health department in your area. They will try to find the animal so it can be tested for rabies.

If the animal control agency or health department can't find the animal that bit you, if the animal shows signs of rabies after the bite, or if a test shows that the animal has rabies, your doctor will probably want you to get a series of rabies shots (also called postexposure prophylaxis). You need to get the first shot as soon as possible after the bite occurs. After you receive the first shot, your doctor will give you five more shots over a 28-day period.

Snakebites: Reducing Your Risk

Reprinted with permission from "Snakebites: Reducing Your Risk," September 2000, updated December 2006, http://familydoctor.org/online/famdocen/home/healthy/ firstaid/bites/153.html. Copyright © 2006 American Academy of Family Physicians. All Rights Reserved.

How can I avoid snakebites?

Snakes are most active in the spring, early summer and fall. Most snakebites occur between April and October, when weather is warm and outdoor activities are popular. Although most snakes are not poisonous, there are several kinds of snakes in the United States that are. These include rattlesnakes, copperheads, cottonmouths, and coral snakes. Each year, approximately 8,000 venomous snakebites occur in the United States. Here are some things you can do to reduce your risk of snakebite:

- Regularly trim hedges, keep your lawn mowed and remove brush from your yard and any nearby vacant lots. This will reduce the number of places where snakes like to live.

- Don't allow children to play in vacant, weed-infested lots.
- Always use tongs when moving firewood, brush, or lumber. This will safely expose any snakes that may be hidden underneath.
- When moving through areas with tall grass and weeds, always poke at the ground ahead of you with a long stick or pole to scare any snakes away.
- Wear loose, long pants and tall boots when working or walking in areas where snakes are likely to be.
- Never handle snakes, even dead ones. If you see a snake, slowly back away from it.
- Always sleep on a cot when camping in snake-infested areas.
- Be aware of snakes if you are swimming or wading in rivers, lakes, or other water such as flooding.
- Learn to identify poisonous snakes and avoid them.

What are the signs of a snakebite?

You may not always know you were bitten by a snake, especially if you were bitten in water or tall grass. Signs and symptoms of a snakebite may include the following:

- Two puncture marks at the wound
- Redness or swelling around the wound
- Severe pain
- Nausea and vomiting
- Labored breathing
- Fever-like symptoms such as sweating
- Numbness or tingling
- Blurred vision
- Diarrhea
- Fainting
- Convulsions
- Rapid pulse

What should I do if I get a snakebite?

A bite from a poisonous snake is a medical emergency. If you or someone else gets bitten by a snake, get help immediately.

What to do if you get bitten by a snake:

- Remain calm and call for help.
- If you are alone, try to get to the nearest hospital as soon as you can.
- Restrict movement as much as possible and try to keep the wound below the level of your heart. This will reduce the spread of venom.
- Take off any jewelry or tight clothing near the bite before swelling starts.
- Try to remember what the snake looked like: its color, shape, and markings. This will help with your treatment.
- Cover the bite with a clean, dry bandage.

What not to do if you get bitten by a snake:

- Never apply ice to the snakebite or soak the wound in water.
- Never cut the place that has been bitten.
- Never try to suck the venom out of the snakebite.
- Never apply a tourniquet or try to stop blood flow to or from the snakebite.
- Never try to pick up or trap the snake.
- Do not drink alcohol to relieve the pain of a snakebite.
- Do not drink caffeinated beverages such as coffee or colas after you've been bitten by a snake.

Chapter 9

Bleeding

Dealing With Bleeding

If you need to give first aid to someone who is bleeding check through D.R.A.B.C.:

- **D**anger: Make sure you and your friend are in a safe place for you to help them.
- **R**esponse: Try to make your friend respond by gently tapping them. If they do not respond they may be unconscious and need additional medical assistance.
- **A**irway: Tilt back your friend's head to open the airway and check if there is anything in their mouth that needs to be removed.
- **B**reathing: Check if your friend is breathing by watching their stomach or putting the back of your hand above their mouth to try and feel air movement.
- **C**irculation: Check your friend's pulse either on the neck or wrist.

If you are in a safe place and your friend is breathing then the next thing you look for is bleeding.

About This Chapter: "First Aid: Bleeding," reprinted with permission. © 2006 Children, Youth and Women's Health Service, Government of South Australia (www.cyh.com).

Heavy Or Major Bleeding

If your friend is bleeding a lot, the first step for you as a first-aider is to stop the bleeding.

1. Get your friend to press hard on that place with her hand. If your friend is not able to stop the bleeding herself then:

2. Press hard with your hand on the wound. Cover your hand if you can (with a glove or clean plastic bag), and press hard on the wound with your hand. If you can't find anything to cover your hand, still try to stop the bleeding by pressing hard with your hand on the wound. Get a clean pad of material like paper towels, clean tissues, a clean hanky (ironing will have killed any germs), scarf, tea towel, or even your jumper, take away the hand which is stopping the bleeding and use the pad to press hard on the wound.

3. Try to lift up the part of the body that is bleeding to slow down the bleeding. (Don't lift it up if it hurts too much. If there are broken bones this could really hurt your friend.) You can get your friend to hold up the injured arm or if it's her leg you could lift her feet and rest them on your knees.

4. Put another pad on top of the first if the blood is coming through. (Don't take the first pad away.)

5. When bleeding stops, keep the pad on and use a bandage to hold it in place.

6. Get help. Send one of the people around you to get help, so that you can stay with your friend. Use a mobile phone if you have one (call 000 in Australia or 911 in the United States).

7. Talk to your friend all the time telling her what you are doing. Then she won't be scared.

8. Keep your friend warm.

9. If she seems to go to sleep she may be unconscious—start DRABC.

> ♣ **It's A Fact!!**
> Blood can carry diseases in it so be careful.
>
> - Try to wash your hands before and after helping someone.
> - Use plastic gloves if you have them.
> - Cover cuts and scratches on your hands if you don't have gloves.
> - Help your friend to deal with the bleeding if she can.

Bleeding

Light Or Minor Bleeding

With a small cut or a wound that is not bleeding much there are three important steps for you to take.

1. Wash the wound with water, (putting it under a running tap can be a good way of cleaning it).
2. Try to get any dirt out of it using water with soap or a bit of disinfectant. Use cotton wool, clean tissues or paper towels, or clean cloth.
3. Cover the wound with a clean dressing.

If you cannot get the dirt out, you will need to see a doctor as dirt inside a wound can cause an infection.

Some kids feel really scared when they see their own blood so keep telling your friend what you are doing and not to be afraid.

Objects In Wounds

Sometimes kids can hurt themselves by falling onto something that sticks into them. Like a piece of broken glass.

Don't pull out the glass or whatever else that is stuck in the wound.

You can stop heavy bleeding by:

- pressing around the wound but not on it.
- putting a pad of clean material around the object and bandaging it in place.
- getting help from a doctor or nurse.

Always talk to an injured friend and ask her to move her body by herself if she can. How would you like someone to grab your sore arm or leg and hold it up in the air without any warning? OUCH!

Nosebleeds

Some people often have nosebleeds and they know how to deal with them. If you, or your friend, don't normally have nose bleeds then here is what you do.

- Sit with your head forward, looking down at the ground.
- Pinch the soft part of the nose together for about ten minutes.
- Putting a cold pack, or ice in a cloth on the back of the neck and forehead can help sometimes, but it is not usually needed.
- When it stops, clean up the mess (put the blood stained tissues into a bin yourself, so that others don't have to handle your blood).
- Your nose will probably feel blocked with blood, and you will want to blow the blood out. Try not to sniff or blow your nose for at least 30 minutes.
- If it doesn't stop keep pinching the soft part of the nose together. Get some more ice or a colder cold pack and hold it on for another 10 minutes.
- Sucking a piece of ice may help (and at least it helps take the taste of blood out of your mouth).
- Get help if the nose is still bleeding after 20 minutes.

Answering Your Questions

Why is it important to look after your hands when you are helping someone who is hurt?

Washing your hands before you help is so that dirt on your hands does not get into the wound. Washing after helping is to clean off any blood that has gotten onto your hands.

Wearing plastic gloves or putting a plastic bag over your hands can protect them too.

If you have a cut, cover it with a waterproof dressing if you can.

> ♣ **It's A Fact!!**
>
> **Dr. Kim Says**
>
> "Seeing blood, especially your own, can be a bit scary. So, if you are helping a friend who is bleeding try to stay calm so that she doesn't get scared. Talk to your friend while you are giving first aid and remember to keep yourself safe by washing your hands carefully with soap after you have finished helping her. If you get someone else's blood onto your hands do not panic! It is very unlikely that this will cause you to be sick, but talk to your doctor if this is worrying you."

Bleeding

What if there is no one to send for help and you don't have a mobile phone?

If there is no one else around, try to stop the bleeding, and go for help when the bleeding stops. If you cannot stop the bleeding and you cannot get help unless you leave your friend, go for help, but get back to your friend as soon as you can.

I have heard that there is a 'blood rule' in sport. What is it and what does it mean?

The "Blood Rule": Most sports have adopted a "rule" which must be followed if a player is wounded during a game because of concerns about spread of blood borne infections. The following is the "Blood Rule" from the Australian Rules Football Rules of the Game (point 1.13).

"A player who is bleeding or who has blood on himself or his uniform is required to leave the ground, at the request of the umpire and have the problem seen to. The player will not be allowed to return until the bleeding has ceased and any blood has been completely removed. This player can be inter-changed off the ground, or the umpire can call a halt to play while the player is seen to. The first option is that most commonly used."

As well as removing all blood, a waterproof dressing should be applied so that if bleeding starts again, it cannot get onto any other player.

Note: If the injury is serious, it would be best for the player not to return to the game. The health of the injured player should come first.

Chapter 10

Burns

Thermal Burns

What are thermal burns?

Thermal burns are burns to the skin caused by any external heat source. This may be in the form of a naked flame from an open fireplace or house fire, a scald from steam, hot or molten liquid, or via direct contact with a hot object such as a hot oven rack or hot cooking pan.

Other types of burns include radiation burns (sunburn from the sun's ultraviolet rays), chemical burns, and electrical burns.

How are thermal burns classified?

To understand the nature and classification of thermal burns it is necessary to have a brief understanding of how skin is made up. Basically, skin consists of an outer layer called the epidermis and an inner layer called the dermis. The epidermis consists of epithelial cells among which are the pigment-containing cells called melanocytes, which absorb some of the potentially dangerous UV rays in sunlight. The epidermis does not contain

---

About This Chapter: This chapter includes "Thermal Burns," © 2008 New Zealand Dermatological Society; and "Chemical Burns," © 2007 New Zealand Dermatological Society. This information is reprinted with the permission from DermNet, the website of the New Zealand Dermatological Society. Visit www.dermnet.org.nz for patient information on numerous skin conditions and their treatment.

Table 10.1. Burn Classifications

Classification	Signs And Symptoms
Superficial or first degree burn	Involves only the epidermis skin layer
	May be painful, red and warm, area turns white when touched, no blisters, moist
Partial thickness or second degree burn	Involves the epidermis and some portion of the dermis
	Depending on the how much of the dermis is affected the burn is further broken down into superficial or deep
	Superficial partial thickness burns are usually painful, red, moist, with blisters, hair still intact
	Deep partial thickness burns may or may not be painful (nerve endings destroyed), may be moist or dry (sweat glands destroyed), hair is usually gone
Full thickness or third degree burn	Most severe burn and involves all layers of skin—epidermis and dermis
	Nerve endings, small blood vessels, hair follicles, sweat glands are all destroyed
	Subcutaneous fat tissue, muscle and bone may also be involved in very severe burns
	Burns are painless with no sensation to touch, skin is pearly white or charred, dry, and may appear leathery

Source: © 2008 New Zealand Dermatological Society.

any blood vessels but is nourished via the blood vessels located in the dermis. Hence, the dermis is richly supplied with blood vessels, lymphatic vessels, and nerves. It also contains hair follicles, sebaceous glands, and sweat glands. Lying below the dermis is the hypodermis or subcutaneous fat tissue. This is not part of the skin but attaches the skin to underlying bone and muscle as well as supplying it with blood vessels and nerves.

Traditionally thermal injuries were classified as first, second, or third degree burns. Nowadays many doctors describe burns according to their thickness (superficial, partial, and full). The signs and symptoms experienced by a burn victim depend largely on the severity of the burn and the number of layers of skin that are affected.

What is the management of thermal burns?

The management of thermal burns involves several key steps:

Evaluation Of The Burn Patient: Evaluating the total well-being of the burn patient is of paramount importance, particularly in patients with large burns. The primary aim is to ensure airway support, gas exchange, and circulatory stability is achieved and maintained. Secondarily, a detailed history should be obtained from the patient to determine how the burn injury occurred. This may give clues for further examination, for example, suspected carbon monoxide poisoning in individuals injured in structural fires.

Evaluation Of The Burn Wound: Evaluation of the burn wound itself should only occur once the patient has been stabilized. The extent and depth of the burn will help guide decisions regarding wound care, inpatient or outpatient care, and monitoring.

♣ **It's A Fact!!**

Extent Of Burn

- Estimates the size of the burn
- Rules of Nines is a tool used to determine the amount of surface area burned (it basically divides the surface area of the body into sections, each roughly 9%)

Depth Of Burn

- Estimates the depth of the burn (what layers of skin are affected)
- Equates to the classification of burns as described
- Estimating the depth of a burn is difficult and often burns are underestimated in depth on initial examination

Source: © 2008 New Zealand Dermatological Society.

♣ It's A Fact!!

Preventing Gasoline Burns

Gasoline Use

- DO remember that gasoline should only be used to fill the gasoline tank of a car, motorcycle, lawn mower, etc. Gasoline's only use is to fuel an engine.

- DO keep in mind that a spark, flame or other source of heat can ignite gasoline vapors, even from many feet away.

- DON'T use gasoline to light a barbecue grill or use it anywhere near a barbecue grill.

- DON'T use gasoline to start or accelerate any kind of fire.

- DON'T use gasoline as a solvent or cleaner.

- DON'T experiment with gasoline in any way. A few minutes of experimentation could result in a lifetime of painful surgeries, disfiguring scars, or even death.

- DON'T sniff or huff gasoline; it can cause brain damage or death.

Handling Gasoline

- DO handle gasoline responsibly at all times and only under adult supervision.

- DO remember that an engine that is still warm can ignite gasoline vapors. Gasoline should only be added when an engine is completely cool.

- DON'T allow younger children to touch gasoline or a gasoline container under any circumstances.

- DON'T handle gasoline near a flame source, such as matches, lighters, or pilot lights on stoves and water heaters.

- DON'T handle gasoline indoors.

- DON'T siphon gasoline by mouth. It is harmful or fatal if swallowed.

- DON'T induce vomiting if gasoline is swallowed. Instead, seek immediate medical attention.

Storing Gasoline

- DO store gasoline only in an approved gasoline container.
- DO store gasoline, or ask your parents to store it, in a well-ventilated outside storage area that is not attached to your home, such as a shed or garage, preferably in a locked cabinet. Be sure there are no ignition sources nearby.
- DO make sure gasoline containers are out of reach of younger siblings or children.
- DO keep only the minimum amount of gasoline required (generally, no more than a gallon).
- DON'T store gasoline in a glass jar, milk jug, or any other non-approved container.
- DON'T keep gasoline anywhere inside a home or vehicle.
- DON'T store gasoline near a source of heat or sparks, such as a hot water heater, furnace, clothes dryer, or any appliance that uses a pilot light or may cause a spark.

About Gasoline Containers

- DO remind your parents to check gasoline containers for compliance with the ASTM F852 standard, which establishes performance requirements for portable gasoline containers intended for reuse by consumers. This compliance is indicated in writing on either side or the underside of all approved plastic gasoline containers.
- DON'T put anything other than gasoline in a gasoline container.
- DON'T drink anything out of a gasoline container.

Source: "Burn Awareness Week: Preventing Gasoline Burns—Important Information for 'Tweens' and 'Teens.'" © 2008 Shriners Hospitals for Children (www.shrinershq.org). Reprinted with permission.

Identifying And Treating Burn Wound Infections: Prompt diagnosis of infection of the burn wound is important to prevent further complication. Two burn wound infections often encountered are:

- **Burn Wound Cellulitis:** Manifests as progressive reddening, swelling, and pain in the uninjured skin around a wound, seen in the first few days after burning. *Streptococcus pyogenes* is the causative bacteria and infection usually responds to penicillin.

- **Invasive Burn Wound Infection:** Rapid growth of bacteria in burn eschar that go on to invade the underlying healthy tissues. A change in color, new drainage, and sometimes a foul or sickly sweet odor are indicative of infection. *Pseudomonas* and other gram-negative bacteria are the common causative agents. These infections can be life threatening and usually require combined treatment with surgery and antibiotics.

Managing The Burn Wound: Any serious burns should be referred to a specialized burns unit, particularly those involving face, hands, and genitalia. For less serious burns, management may be in the outpatient or inpatient setting.

The main treatment aims of burn wound management are:

- Carefully monitor wound;
- Keep wounds clean;
- Prevent the wound drying out;
- Manage secondary infection.

Commonly used topical antibacterials include 1% silver sulfadiazine cream, 0.5% silver nitrate solution and mafenide acetate 10% cream.

Chemical Burns

What are chemical burns?

Chemical burns are burns to internal or external organs of the body caused mainly by chemical substances that are strong acids or bases (also known as alkalies). Chemical burns are usually the result of an accident and can occur

Burns

in the home, at school, or more commonly, at work, particularly in manufacturing plants that use large quantities of chemicals.

Very mild chemical burns result in irritant contact dermatitis.

What causes chemical burns?

The main cause of chemical burns is from contact with strong acids or bases. The strength of acids and bases is defined by the pH scale, which ranges from 1 to 14. A very strong acid has a pH of 1 and may cause a severe burn. A very strong base has a pH of 14 and may also cause a severe burn. A substance with a pH of 7 is considered neutral and does not burn. Chemical burns from acids or bases are also referred to as caustic burns.

Table 10.2 lists some common products containing chemical substances that may potentially cause chemical burns.

What are the signs and symptoms of chemical burns?

The signs and symptoms of a chemical burn depend on several factors, including:

- pH of the agent;
- concentration of the agent;
- length of contact time;
- amount of agent involved;
- physical form of the agent (solid, liquid, gas);
- site of contact (for example, eye, skin, mucous membrane);
- whether swallowed or inhaled;
- whether or not skin is intact.

The swallowing of solid pellets of alkaline substances highlights the importance of these factors. The solid pellets will sit in the stomach for a longer period, thus more severe burns sustained. Another important factor is concentrated forms of some acids and bases generate a large amount of heat when diluted, this results not only in chemical burns but thermal burns too.

Table 10.2. Common Products That May Potentially Cause Chemical Burns

Common Acids	Products
Sulfuric acid, concentration ranging from 8% to almost pure acid	Toilet bowl cleaners Drain cleaners Metal cleaners Car battery fluid Fertilizer manufacturing
Nitric acid	Used in engraving, metal refining, electroplating, and fertilizer manufacturing
Hydrofluoric acid, a weak acid and in a dilute form does not burn or cause pain on contact	Rust removers Tire cleaners Tile cleaners Glass etching Dental work Refrigerant
Hydrochloric acid, concentrations range 5–44%	Toilet bowl cleaners Metal cleaners Swimming pool cleaners Dye manufacturing Metal refining
Phosphoric acid	Metal cleaners Rustproofing Disinfectants, detergents Fertilizer manufacturing

Common Bases	Products
Sodium hydroxide and potassium hydroxide, depending on the concentration may be very corrosive	Drain cleaners Oven cleaners Denture cleaners
Sodium and calcium hypochlorite	Household bleach Pool chlorinating solution
Ammonia	Cleaners and detergents used in the dilute form is not highly corrosive Gaseous anhydrous ammonia used in fertilizing manufacturing can cause severe burns
Phosphates	Many household detergents and cleaners

Source: © 2007 New Zealand Dermatological Society.

Burns

Some signs and symptoms of chemical burns include:

- Redness, irritation, or burning at the site of contact;
- Pain or numbness at the site of contact;
- Formation of black dead skin (eschar)—this occurs particularly with acid chemical burns as they produce a coagulation necrosis by denaturing proteins;
- Deep tissue injury to the skin is caused by alkali chemical burns as they produce a liquefaction necrosis that involves denaturing of proteins as well as saponification of fats;
- Vision changes or complete loss of vision if chemicals get into the eyes.

In severe chemical burns where the agent has been swallowed, inhaled, or absorbed into the bloodstream, the following systemic symptoms may occur:

- Cough or shortness of breath
- Low blood pressure
- Faintness, weakness, dizziness
- Headache
- Muscle twitching or seizures
- Cardiac arrest or irregular heartbeat

What is the management of chemical burns?

Basic first aid should be administered as soon as a chemical burn has occurred. This should include removal of contaminated clothing and prompt irrigation of the affected area with copious amounts of water. Wash for at least 20 minutes, taking care not to allow runoff to contact unaffected areas. It has been shown that irrigation received within 10 minutes of the burn reduces the severity of the wound and time of stay in hospital.

Chemical burns involving elemental metals (lithium, potassium, sodium and magnesium) should not be irrigated with water as this can result in a chemical reaction that causes burns to worsen. These types of chemical burns should be soaked with mineral oil while waiting for medical attention.

People with minor chemical burns do not require hospitalization. For more severe burns patients should receive treatment as for a typical thermal burn patient. In some situations an antidote may be given to counteract the offending chemical agent.

The main treatment aims of burn wound management are:

- Carefully monitor wound;

✔ **Quick Tip**

Respond

There are several types of burn injuries. In the event of any burn injury, it is imperative that medical attention is sought immediately. The procedures below can be followed until medical help arrives:

Thermal burns are caused by contact with an open flame or other source of high heat, including appliances, steam or hot liquids.

- Put out any fire or flame or stop contact with steam, liquid or object.
- Remove hot or burned clothing, if possible.
- Cool injured area with running water within 30 seconds.
- Stop any bleeding.
- Cover burned area with sterile pad or clean sheet
- Attempt to maintain victims body temperature.
- Seek medical help.

Chemical burns are caused by contact with strong acids or bases. Household products such as bleach, concrete mix, and pool chlorinators are among the most common sources of chemical burns.

- Flush affected skin with cool, running water for 20 minutes or more. If the chemical is a powder, brush it off the skin before flushing.
- Seek medical help. Even if the area is washed, the chemical may have penetrated.
- Contact poison control or your local emergency room.

Burns

- Keep wounds clean;
- Prevent the wound drying out;
- Manage secondary infection.

Commonly used topical antibacterials include 1% silver sulfadiazine cream, 0.5% silver nitrate solution and mafenide acetate 10% cream.

Electrical burns occur when strong electrical currents pass through the body. These burns may appear minor, but the damage can extend deep into the tissues beneath the skin.

- Look first and do not touch the victim, as the person may still in contact with the electrical source.
- Pull the plug or shut off any electrical current.
- Check the victim's breathing. If breathing has stopped or you suspect the airway is blocked, begin CPR (cardiopulmonary resuscitation).
- Cover affected areas using a sterile gauze bandage or clean cloth. Do not use a blanket or towel as fluffy fibers can be irritating.
- Seek medical help.

For any burn:

- Never apply lotions, ointments, or creams to the affected area.
- Never use adhesive dressings.
- Never break blisters.

Source: Excerpted from "Burn Injuries," © Shriners Hospitals for Children (www.shrinershq.org). Reprinted with permission.

Chapter 11

Broken Bones

A broken or cracked bone is known as a fracture. Fractures can affect any bone in the body.

Bones can fracture in a number of different ways. A fracture may be a straight break across the bone (transverse fracture), slanting (oblique fracture), or winding (spiral fracture). The break may run along the shaft of the bone (longitudinal fracture), or the bone may be shattered into pieces (comminuted fracture). Young bone is softer and more able to bend than adult bone, so children's bones often fracture on one side but bend on the other. This is known as a greenstick fracture.

An avulsion fracture is when a piece of bone detaches from the main bone, usually because of being torn away by the tendon that attaches a muscle to a bone. A fracture in which the bone collapses is called a compression fracture. Compression fractures usually affect the spongy bone found in the spine.

A fracture in which the skin around the bone has not been broken is called a simple or closed fracture. If the ends of the bone break through the skin, or there is a wound that leads to the fractured bone, it is called a compound or open fracture. In a compound fracture the bone is open to infection, so this type of fracture is more serious.

About This Chapter: NHS Direct Online. © 2007 Crown copyright material is reproduced with the permission of the Controller of HMSO and Queen's Printer for Scotland.

A complicated fracture is one in which there is injury to other nearby structures, such as major blood vessels and nerves. A fracture-dislocation occurs when a joint becomes dislocated and there is also a fracture of one of the bones of the joint.

After a fracture, the broken fragments of bone normally separate from each other. However, sometimes one fragment of bone can be driven into another. This is known as an impacted fracture.

Symptoms

The symptoms of a fracture depend on the bone affected and the severity of the injury, but can include:

- pain and swelling;
- bruising or discolored skin around the bone or joint;
- the limb or part of the body being bent at an unusual angle (angulation);
- being unable to move or put weight on the injured limb or part; and
- a grinding or grating sensation or sound in the bone or joint (crepitus).

A person who has fractured a bone may appear pale and clammy and may feel faint, dizzy, or sick. This will normally be due to the pain. However, when large bones such as the pelvis or femur (the bone in the thigh) break, there can be internal bleeding from the bone and this can cause similar symptoms.

Unless it is essential to do so, you should not move a person with a fractured limb until a splint has been applied by a doctor or paramedic to prevent movement of the injured part and the joints above and below the fracture.

If you think you may have fractured a bone you should seek medical help immediately.

Causes

Bones are rigid, but they do bend a little when a force is applied to them. When the force stops the bone returns to its original shape.

Broken Bones

Healthy bones are very strong and are normally able to withstand large forces. However, if the force is too great the bone will crack or break. Bones can also fracture as a result of repeated small stresses or strains. This type of fracture is known as a stress fracture.

Fractures are usually caused by physical injury—for example, from an accident such as a fall or a car crash. Excessive force will fracture any bone, but a bone will fracture more easily if it has already been generally weakened by a disease such as osteoporosis (which makes bones become thin and weak), or weakened in a specific place by a tumor or cyst. This type of fracture is called a pathological fracture

Treatment

Treatment of a fracture starts with lining up (aligning) the ends of the broken bone properly, so that the natural healing process can begin. Aligning the broken bone is known as reducing the fracture.

Fracture reduction is normally done under general anesthetic. It may be done without surgery by manipulating or pulling the injured area (traction), or surgery may be used to re-align bones or bone fragments. Transverse fractures are often harder to align and immobilize than more serious oblique or spiral fractures.

> ♣ **It's A Fact!!**
> **Diagnosis**
>
> Fractures are usually first diagnosed from their symptoms, a physical examination, and by taking a patient history. The diagnosis will be confirmed with an x-ray.
>
> Some types of fracture are difficult to see and it may take a series of x-rays or a magnetic resonance imaging (MRI) or computed tomography (CT) scan to identify the fracture.

Once aligned, the ends of the broken bone must be held in the proper position while they heal. This is known as immobilization. There are various methods used to immobilize fractured bones, including:

- plaster, plastic, or resin casts;
- steel plates and screws;
- internal steel rods (intramedullary nails) for long bones; and

- external fixing devices consisting of a steel beam, to which are attached at least four steel pins (fixators) that pass into the bone above and below the fracture site.

Immobilization may be necessary for between two and eight weeks, depending on the bone involved and on whether there are complications such as infection or damage to the blood supply to the bone.

Most broken bones heal successfully once they have been aligned correctly and immobilized. During the healing process, special cells (osteoclasts) remove damaged bone splinters, while other cells (osteoblasts) form a tissue called a callus around the injured area. New bone cells start to grow on either side of the fracture and towards each other until the fracture is closed. Over time, the callus is smoothed off and eventually the bone returns to its normal thickness.

Compound and complicated fractures often require surgery to repair the damage to the tissues that surround the bone or joint.

The time it takes for a broken bone to heal fully depends on the bone affected and the type of fracture. In some cases, physiotherapy may be needed to help build up strength and restore mobility in the injured area.

Some fractures refuse to heal or are slow to do so. In these cases, a treatment called physical field therapy may help. Ultrasound or pulsed electromagnetic energy is applied to the area of the break through a device placed on the surface of the skin.

Prevention

To grow, develop, and maintain healthy bones, it is important that you have enough calcium in your diet. Good sources of calcium include milk, cheese, and yogurt. Vitamin D helps the body to absorb calcium—you can find it in margarine and oily fish.

Because of the way bones are made, they get stronger and denser with regular exercise. It is particularly important that older people remain active, as this will help to reduce their risk of fractures.

Broken Bones

The female hormone estrogen regulates the use of calcium in a woman's body. After the menopause, women produce far less estrogen, making calcium regulation more difficult. This means that it is particularly important that women make their bones as strong as possible before the menopause.

> ♣ **It's A Fact!!**
> **Complications**
>
> A compound fracture can lead to infection of the bone or bone marrow. In some cases this infection can progress to a chronic infection called osteomyelitis, requiring treatment with antibiotics and careful management in hospital.
>
> If the bones in a fracture refuse to join up again, or if they take a particularly long time to do so, the bone may lose its blood supply and die. This is known as avascular necrosis. In some cases, surgery may be needed if the fracture refuses to join up.
>
> Fractures near or through joints may result in the joint becoming permanently stiff or unable to bend properly.

Chapter 12
Spinal Cord Injuries

What is a spinal cord injury?

Although the hard bones of the spinal column protect the soft tissues of the spinal cord, vertebrae can still be broken or dislocated in a variety of ways and cause traumatic injury to the spinal cord. Injuries can occur at any level of the spinal cord. The segment of the cord that is injured and the severity of the injury will determine which body functions are compromised or lost. Because the spinal cord acts as the main information pathway between the brain and the rest of the body, a spinal cord injury can have significant physiological consequences.

Catastrophic falls, being thrown from a horse or through a windshield, or any kind of physical trauma that crushes and compresses the vertebrae in the neck can cause irreversible damage at the cervical level of the spinal cord and below. Paralysis of most of the body including the arms and legs, called quadriplegia, is the likely result. Automobile accidents are often responsible for spinal cord damage in the middle back (the thoracic or lumbar area), which can cause paralysis of the lower trunk and lower extremities, called paraplegia.

Other kinds of injuries that directly penetrate the spinal cord, such as gunshot or knife wounds, can either completely or partially sever the spinal cord and create life-long disabilities.

> About This Chapter: Excerpted from "Spinal Cord Injury: Hope Through Research," National Institute of Neurological Disorders and Stroke, NIH Pub. No. 03-160, updated December 11, 2007.

Most injuries to the spinal cord don't completely sever it. Instead, an injury is more likely to cause fractures and compression of the vertebrae, which then crush and destroy the axons, extensions of nerve cells that carry signals up and down the spinal cord between the brain and the rest of the body. An injury to the spinal cord can damage a few, many, or almost all of these axons. Some injuries will allow almost complete recovery. Others will result in complete paralysis.

How does the spinal cord work?

To understand what can happen as the result of a spinal cord injury, it helps to know the anatomy of the spinal cord and its normal functions.

Spine Anatomy: The soft, jelly-like spinal cord is protected by the spinal column. The spinal column is made up of 33 bones called vertebrae, each with a circular opening similar to the hole in a donut. The bones are stacked one on top of the other and the spinal cord runs through the hollow channel created by the holes in the stacked bones.

The vertebrae can be organized into sections, and are named and numbered from top to bottom according to their location along the backbone:

- Cervical vertebrae (1–7) located in the neck
- Thoracic vertebrae (1–12) in the upper back (attached to the ribcage)
- Lumbar vertebrae (1–5) in the lower back
- Sacral vertebrae (1–5) in the hip area
- Coccygeal vertebrae (1–4 fused) in the tailbone

Although the hard vertebrae protect the soft spinal cord from injury most of the time, the spinal column is not all hard bone. Between the vertebrae are discs of semi-rigid cartilage, and in the narrow spaces between them are passages through which the spinal nerves exit to the rest of the body. These are places where the spinal cord is vulnerable to direct injury.

The spinal cord is also organized into segments and named and numbered from top to bottom. Each segment marks where spinal nerves emerge

Spinal Cord Injuries

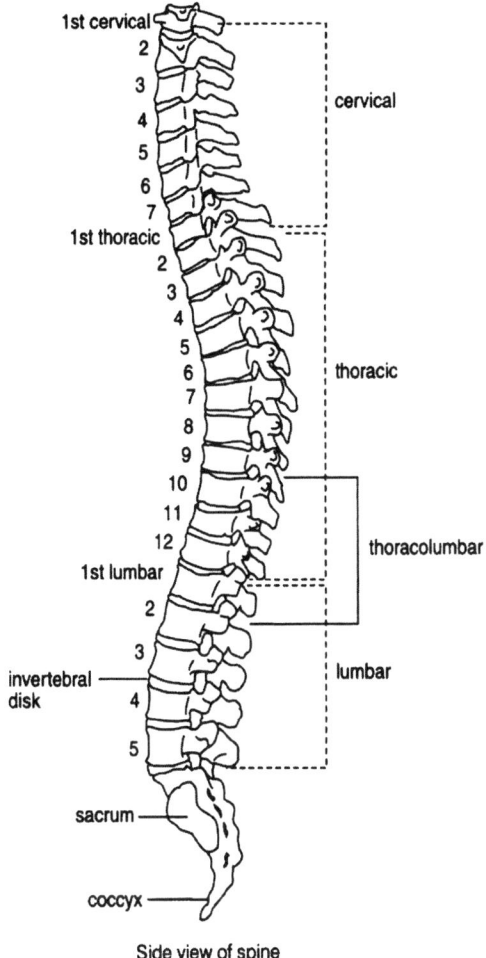

Figure 12.1. Side view of spine (Source: From "Questions and Answers about Scoliosis in Children and Adolescents," NIAMS, July 2001.)

from the cord to connect to specific regions of the body. Locations of spinal cord segments do not correspond exactly to vertebral locations, but they are roughly equivalent.

- Cervical spinal nerves (C1 to C8) control signals to the back of the head, the neck and shoulders, the arms and hands, and the diaphragm.
- Thoracic spinal nerves (T1 to T12) control signals to the chest muscles, some muscles of the back, and parts of the abdomen.

- Lumbar spinal nerves (L1 to L5) control signals to the lower parts of the abdomen and the back, the buttocks, some parts of the external genital organs, and parts of the leg.
- Sacral spinal nerves (S1 to S5) control signals to the thighs and lower parts of the legs, the feet, most of the external genital organs, and the area around the anus.
- The single coccygeal nerve carries sensory information from the skin of the lower back.

The ascending sensory tracts transmit sensory signals from the skin, extremities, and internal organs that enter at specific segments of the spinal cord. Most of these signals are then relayed to the brain. The spinal cord also contains neuronal circuits that control reflexes and repetitive movements, such as walking, which can be activated by incoming sensory signals without input from the brain.

The circumference of the spinal cord varies depending on its location. It is larger in the cervical and lumbar areas because these areas supply the nerves to the arms and upper body and the legs and lower body, which require the most intense muscular control and receive the most sensory signals.

The ratio of white matter to grey matter also varies at each level of the spinal cord. In the cervical segment, which is located in the neck, there is a large amount of white matter because at this level there are many axons going to and from the brain and the rest of the spinal cord below. In lower segments, such as the sacral, there is less white matter because most ascending axons have not yet entered the cord, and most descending axons have contacted their targets along the way.

To pass between the vertebrae, the axons that link the spinal cord to the muscles and the rest of the body are bundled into 31 pairs of spinal nerves, each pair with a sensory root and a motor root that make connections within the grey matter. Two pairs of nerves—a sensory and motor pair on either side of the cord—emerge from each segment of the spinal cord.

The functions of these nerves are determined by their location in the spinal cord. They control everything from body functions such as breathing, sweating, digestion, and elimination, to gross and fine motor skills, as well as sensations in the arms and legs.

Spinal Cord Injuries

What are the immediate treatments for spinal cord injury?

The outcome of any injury to the spinal cord depends upon the number of axons that survive: the higher the number of normally functioning axons, the less the amount of disability. Consequently, the most important consideration when moving people to a hospital or trauma center is preventing further injury to the spine and spinal cord.

Spinal cord injury isn't always obvious. Any injury that involves the head (especially with trauma to the front of the face), pelvic fractures, penetrating injuries in the area of the spine, or injuries that result from falling from heights should be suspect for spinal cord damage.

> **What's It Mean?**
>
> Myelin: A structure of cell membranes that forms a sheath around axons, insulating them and speeding conduction of nerve impulses.
>
> Sacral: Refers to the part of the spine in the hip area.

Until imaging of the spine is done at an emergency or trauma center, people who might have spinal cord injury should be cared for as if any significant movement of the spine could cause further damage. They are usually transported in a recumbent (lying down) position, with a rigid collar and backboard immobilizing the spine.

Spinal cord injuries are classified as either complete or incomplete, depending on how much cord width is injured. An incomplete injury means that the ability of the spinal cord to convey messages to or from the brain is not completely lost. People with incomplete injuries retain some motor or sensory function below the injury.

A complete injury is indicated by a total lack of sensory and motor function below the level of injury.

How does a spinal cord injury affect the rest of the body?

People who survive a spinal cord injury will most likely have medical complications such as chronic pain and bladder and bowel dysfunction, along with an increased susceptibility to respiratory and heart problems. Successful recovery depends upon how well these chronic conditions are handled day to day.

- **Breathing:** Any injury to the spinal cord at or above the C3, C4, and C5 segments, which supply the phrenic nerves leading to the diaphragm, can stop breathing.

- **Pneumonia:** Respiratory complications, primarily as a result of pneumonia, are a leading cause of death in people with spinal cord injury.

- **Irregular Heart Beat And Low Blood Pressure:** Spinal cord injuries in the cervical region are often accompanied by blood pressure instability and heart arrhythmias.

- **Blood Clots:** People with spinal cord injuries are at triple the usual risk for blood clots.

- **Spasm:** Many of our reflex movements are controlled by the spinal cord but regulated by the brain. When the spinal cord is damaged, information from the brain can no longer regulate reflex activity. Reflexes may become exaggerated over time, causing spasticity.

- **Autonomic Dysreflexia:** Autonomic dysreflexia is a life-threatening reflex action that primarily affects those with injuries to the neck or upper back. It happens when there is an irritation, pain, or stimulus to the nervous system below the level of injury. The irritated area tries to send a signal to the brain, but since the signal isn't able to get through, a reflex action occurs without the brain's regulation. Unlike spasms that affect muscles, autonomic dysreflexia affects vascular and organ systems controlled by the sympathetic nervous system.

- **Pressure Sores:** Pressure sores (or pressure ulcers) are areas of skin tissue that have broken down because of continuous pressure on the skin. People with paraplegia and quadriplegia are susceptible to pressure sores because they can't move easily on their own.

- **Pain:** People who are paralyzed often have what is called neurogenic pain resulting from damage to nerves in the spinal cord.

- **Bladder And Bowel Problems:** Most spinal cord injuries affect bladder and bowel functions because the nerves that control the involved organs originate in the segments near the lower termination of the spinal cord and are cut off from brain input.

Spinal Cord Injuries

- **Reproductive And Sexual Function:** Spinal cord injury has a greater impact on sexual and reproductive function in men than it does in women. Most spinal cord injured women remain fertile and can conceive and bear children. Depending on the level of injury, men may have problems with erections and ejaculation, and most will have compromised fertility due to decreased motility of their sperm.

How does rehabilitation help people recover from spinal cord injuries?

No two people will experience the same emotions after surviving a spinal cord injury, but almost everyone will feel frightened, anxious, or confused about what has happened. It's common for people to have very mixed feelings: relief that they are still alive, but disbelief at the nature of their disabilities.

Rehabilitation programs combine physical therapies with skill-building activities and counseling to provide social and emotional support. The education and active involvement of the newly injured person and his or her family and friends is crucial.

A rehabilitation team is usually led by a doctor specializing in physical medicine and rehabilitation (called a physiatrist), and often includes social workers, physical and occupational therapists, recreational therapists, rehabilitation nurses, rehabilitation psychologists, vocational counselors, nutritionists, and other specialists. A case-worker or program manager coordinates care.

In the initial phase of rehabilitation, therapists emphasize regaining leg and arm strength since mobility and communication are the two most important areas of function. For some, mobility will only be possible with the assistance of devices such as a walker, leg braces, or a wheelchair. Communication skills, such as writing, typing, and using the telephone, may also require adaptive devices.

Physical therapy includes exercise programs geared toward muscle strengthening. Occupational therapy helps redevelop fine motor skills. Bladder and bowel management programs teach basic toileting routines, and patients also learn techniques for self-grooming. People acquire coping strategies for recurring episodes of spasticity, autonomic dysreflexia, and neurogenic pain.

Vocational rehabilitation begins with an assessment of basic work skills, current dexterity, and physical and cognitive capabilities to determine the likelihood for employment. A vocational rehabilitation specialist then identifies potential work places, determines the type of assistive equipment that will be needed, and helps arrange for a user-friendly workplace. For those whose disabilities prevent them from returning to the workplace, therapists focus on encouraging productivity through participation in activities that provide a sense of satisfaction and self-esteem. This could include educational classes, hobbies, memberships in special interest groups, and participation in family and community events.

Recreation therapy encourages patients to build on their abilities so that they can participate in recreational or athletic activities at their level of mobility. Engaging in recreational outlets and athletics helps those with spinal cord injuries achieve a more balanced and normal lifestyle and also provides opportunities for socialization and self-expression.

> ♣ It's A Fact!!
> ## Can an injured spinal cord be rebuilt?
>
> This is the question that drives basic research in the field of spinal cord injury. As investigators try to understand the underlying biological mechanisms that either inhibit or promote new growth in the spinal cord, they are making surprising discoveries, not just about how neurons and their axons grow in the central nervous system (CNS), but also about why they fail to regenerate after injury in the adult CNS. Understanding the cellular and molecular mechanisms involved in both the working and the damaged spinal cord could point the way to therapies that might prevent secondary damage, encourage axons to grow past injured areas, and reconnect vital neural circuits within the spinal cord and CNS.
>
> There has been successful research in a number of fields that may someday help people with spinal cord injuries. Genetic studies have revealed a number of molecules that encourage axon growth in the developing CNS but prevent it in the adult. Research into embryonic and adult stem cell biology has furthered knowledge about how cells communicate with each other.
>
> Basic research has helped describe the mechanisms involved in the mysterious process of apoptosis, in which large groups of seemingly healthy cells self-destruct. New rehabilitation therapies that retrain neural circuits through forced motion and electrical stimulation of muscle groups are helping injured patients regain lost function.

Chapter 13

Concussions

What Is A Concussion And What Causes It?

The brain is made of soft tissue and is cushioned by spinal fluid. It is encased in the hard, protective skull. When a person gets a head injury, the brain can slosh around inside the skull and even bang against it. This can lead to bruising of the brain, tearing of blood vessels, and injury to the nerves. When this happens, a person can get a concussion—a temporary loss of normal brain function. Most people with concussions recover just fine with appropriate treatment. But it's important to take proper steps if you suspect a concussion because it can be serious.

Concussions and other brain injuries are fairly common. About every 21 seconds, someone in the United States has a serious brain injury. One of the most common reasons people get concussions is through a sports injury. High-contact sports such as football, boxing, and hockey pose a higher risk of head injury, even with the use of protective headgear.

People can also get concussions from falls, car accidents, bike and blading mishaps, and physical violence, such as fighting. Guys are more likely to get

---

About This Chapter: "Concussions," May 2007, reprinted with permission from www.kidshealth.org. Copyright © 2007 The Nemours Foundation. This information was provided by KidsHealth, one of the largest resources online for medically reviewed health information written for parents, kids, and teens. For more articles like this one, visit www.KidsHealth.org, or www.TeensHealth.org.

concussions than girls. However, in certain sports, like soccer, girls have a higher potential for concussion.

What Are The Signs And Symptoms?

The signs of concussion are not always well recognized. And because of that, teens may put themselves at risk for another injury. For example, players may return to a game before they should, or a skateboarder may get back on the board and continue skating, thinking nothing's wrong. That's a problem, because if the brain hasn't healed properly from a concussion and someone gets another brain injury (even if it's with less force), it can be serious.

> ♣ **It's A Fact!!**
> **Heads Up:** People who get repeated head injuries can have permanent brain damage if they try to resume their normal routine too quickly after a concussion.

Repeated injury to the brain can lead to swelling, and sometimes people develop long-term disabilities, or even die, as a result of serious head injuries. So it's really important to recognize and understand the signals of a concussion.

Although we may think of a concussion as someone losing consciousness (passing out), a person can have a concussion and never lose consciousness.

Symptoms of a concussion may include:
- "seeing stars" and feeling dazed, dizzy, or lightheaded;
- memory loss, such as trouble remembering things that happened right before and after the injury;
- nausea or vomiting;
- headaches;
- blurred vision and sensitivity to light;
- slurred speech or saying things that don't make sense;
- difficulty concentrating, thinking, or making decisions;
- difficulty with coordination or balance (such as being unable to catch a ball or other easy tasks);

- feeling anxious or irritable for no apparent reason;
- feeling overly tired.

Different Grades Of Concussion

There are different grades of concussion:

- Someone with a grade 1 concussion can have some of the symptoms listed above, but with no loss of consciousness and with symptoms ending within 15 minutes.
- With a grade 2 concussion, there has been no loss of consciousness but the symptoms last longer than 15 minutes.
- In a grade 3 concussion, the person loses consciousness—even if it's just for a few seconds.

Knowing the different grades is important because how soon a player can safely return to a sports activity is tied to the grade of the concussion:

- With a grade 1 concussion, the player can resume play once symptoms have stopped. However, that player should stop play if he or she gets another head injury.
- A grade 2 concussion requires that a player stop playing and not return to any type of sport or physical activity that could cause a head injury for at least another week.
- Someone with a grade 3 concussion should see a doctor as quickly as possible.

What Do Doctors Do?

If a doctor suspects that someone may have a concussion, he or she will ask about the head injury—such as how it happened and when—and the symptoms. The doctor may ask what seem like silly questions—things like "Who are you?" or "Where are you?" or "What day is it?" and "Who is the president?" Doctors ask these questions to check the person's level of consciousness and memory and concentration abilities.

The doctor will perform a thorough examination of the nervous system, including testing balance, coordination of movement, and reflexes. The doctor

> ✔ **Quick Tip**
> **What should you do if a friend or teammate has a concussion?**
>
> Tell an adult or coach immediately. Even if the concussion seems mild, the player should sit out for the rest of the game. If the symptoms are severe (such as seizures or a very long period of unconsciousness) or they seem to be getting worse, that's an indication of a serious head injury. Get medical help right away.

may ask the patient to do some activity such as running in place for a few minutes to see how well the brain functions after a physical workout.

Sometimes a doctor may order a CT scan (a special brain x-ray) or an MRI (a special non-x-ray brain image) to rule out bleeding or other serious injury involving the brain.

If the concussion isn't serious enough to require hospitalization, the doctor will give instructions on what to do at home, like having someone wake the person up at least once during the night. If a person with a concussion cannot be easily awakened, becomes increasingly confused, or has other symptoms such as vomiting, it may mean there is a more severe problem that requires contacting the doctor again.

The doctor will probably recommend that someone with a concussion take acetaminophen or other aspirin-free medications for headaches. The person also will have to take things easy at school or work.

After A Concussion

After a concussion, the brain needs time to heal. It's really important to wait until all symptoms of a concussion have cleared up before returning to normal activities. The amount of time someone needs to recover depends on how long the symptoms last. Healthy teens can usually resume their normal activities within a few weeks, but each situation is different. A doctor will monitor the person closely to make sure everything's OK.

Concussions

Someone who has had a concussion and has not recovered within a few months is said to have postconcussion syndrome. The person may have the same problems described earlier—such as poor memory, headaches, dizziness, and irritability—but these will last for longer periods of time and may even be permanent.

If someone has continuing problems after a concussion, the doctor may refer him or her to a rehabilitation specialist for additional help.

Can Concussions Be Prevented?

Some accidents can't be avoided. But you can do a lot to prevent a concussion by taking simple precautions:

- Always wear a seat belt in a car. If you drive, be attentive at all times, and obey speed limits, signs, and safe-driving laws to reduce the chances of having an accident. Driving rules and regulations were created to protect everyone. Never use alcohol or other drugs when you're behind the wheel. There's a reason it's illegal: Alcohol and drugs make your reaction time slower and impair your judgment, making you much more likely to have an accident.

- Wearing appropriate headgear and safety equipment when biking, blading, skateboarding, snowboarding or skiing, and playing contact sports can significantly reduce your chances of having a concussion. By wearing a bike helmet, for instance, you can reduce your risk of having a concussion by about 85%.

Taking good care of yourself after a concussion is essential. If you reinjure your brain during the time it is still healing, it will take even more time to completely heal. Each time a person has a concussion, it does additional damage. Having multiple concussions over a period of time has the same effect on a person as being knocked unconscious for several hours.

Preventing concussions is mostly common sense. The best thing you can do to protect your head is to use it.

Chapter 14

Traumatic Brain Injury

What is a traumatic brain injury?

A traumatic brain injury (TBI) is defined as a blow or jolt to the head or a penetrating head injury that disrupts the normal function of the brain. Not all blows or jolts to the head result in a TBI. The severity of such an injury may range from "mild," that is, a brief change in mental status or consciousness to "severe," that is, an extended period of unconsciousness or amnesia after the injury. A TBI can result in short or long-term problems with an individual's ability to function independently, or changes that affect thinking, memory, sensation, language, and emotions.

What are some common signs and symptoms of a TBI?

The signs and symptoms of a TBI can be subtle. Symptoms of a TBI may not appear until days or weeks following the injury or may even be missed as people may look fine even though they may act or feel differently. The following are some common signs and symptoms of a TBI:

- Headaches or neck pain that do not go away
- Difficulty remembering, concentrating, or making decisions

About This Chapter: This chapter begins with excerpts from "Brain Injuries and Mass Casualty Events," Centers for Disease Control and Prevention (CDC), June 2006. Additional information from ThinkFirst National Injury Prevention Foundation is cited separately within the chapter.

- Slowness in thinking, speaking, acting, or reading
- Getting lost or easily confused
- Feeling tired all of the time, having no energy or motivation
- Mood changes (feeling sad or angry for no reason)
- Changes in sleep patterns (sleeping a lot more or having a hard time sleeping)
- Light-headedness, dizziness, or loss of balance
- Urge to vomit (nausea)
- Increased sensitivity to lights, sounds, or distractions
- Blurred vision or eyes that tire easily
- Loss of sense of smell or taste
- Ringing in the ears

> ✔ **Quick Tip**
> If you think you or someone you know has a traumatic brain injury, contact your health care provider. Your health care provider can refer you to a neurologist, neuropsychologist, neurosurgeon, or specialist in rehabilitation (such as a speech pathologist). Getting help soon after the injury by trained specialists may speed your recovery.
>
> Source: CDC, 2006.

Statistics And Prevention

"Injury Prevention," © 2008 ThinkFirst National Injury Prevention Foundation (www.thinkfirst.org). Reprinted with permission.

Death And Injury Statistics

- Traumatic brain injury (TBI) is the number one cause of both death and disability in children and young adults.
- Approximately 5.3 million Americans are currently disabled as a result of a brain injury.
- Every five minutes one person will die and another will become permanently disabled due to a brain injury.
- Approximately 1.5 million Americans sustain a TBI each year.

Traumatic Brain Injury

- It is estimated that TBIs claim more than 50,000 American lives annually.
- 80,000–90,000 individuals suffer long-term disability as a result of a brain injury.
- Falls are the leading cause of brain injuries among the elderly.
- 33–50% of traumatic brain injury victims were intoxicated at the time of the incident, which increases the incidence of death and makes recovery more difficult.

When Injuries Are Most Likely To Occur

- 51% of incidents resulting in brain injury occur on the weekend.
- Most brain injuries take place at night.

Consequences

- 90% of victims' cognitive functions are affected. This includes:
    - Memory loss;
    - Impaired judgment;
    - Difficulty concentrating and completing tasks;
    - Difficulty communicating.
- 61% have decreased neurophysical ability, such as:
    - Seizures;
    - Loss of smell, taste, or vision;
    - Speech impairments;
    - Headaches;
    - Fatigue;
    - Loss of balance.

> ♣ **It's A Fact!!**
> **Who is most likely to incur this type of injury?**
>
> - Only 21.2% of the TBI injuries involved females while 78.8% involved males.
> - Each year, more than 30,000 children suffer permanent disabilities as a result of a brain injury.
> - African American children four and under are 40% more likely to incur a TBI than Caucasian children.
>
> Source: © 2008 ThinkFirst National Injury Prevention Foundation (www.thinkfirst.org).

- 77.5% suffer from psychosocial difficulties including:
    - Depression and mood changes;
    - Anxiousness;
    - Impulsiveness;
    - Self-centered behavior.

Health Costs

- A TBI survivor pays approximately $4 million in their lifetime for healthcare and services.
    - 50% of deaths due to TBI take place within 10 minutes of the incident.

Prevention Tips

- Always wear a Snell (Snell is one of the leaders in helmet safety testing), ANSI (American National Standards Institute) and/or ASTM (American Society for Testing and Materials) certified bicycle helmet and/or protective gear when riding a bicycle, skateboard, or inline skating.
- Always wear a DOT certified motorcycle helmet when riding a motorcycle.
- Always wear a safety belt when driving or riding in a motor vehicle.
- Never drink and drive. Always have a designated driver.
- Always observe and obey speed limits, traffic signs and signals.
- Make sure when playing on a playground that the ground surface is soft and free of debris and rocks.

Still Not Convinced?

In the United States, one person incurs a traumatic brain injury every 21 seconds. This means that in the short time it has taken you to read these facts, approximately 13 people have suffered traumatic brain injuries. Your brain is irreplaceable. It cannot be mended like a broken bone. If you are lucky enough to survive a TBI, any damage that your brain has sustained will

Traumatic Brain Injury

stay with you for life. It has been verified that helmets, safety belts, air bags, and car seats decrease the risk of traumatic brain injury and death. In fact, wearing a bicycle helmet can reduce TBI by 85%. Brain injuries are serious problems with serious consequences, so take the proper precautions to protect yourself. If you don't, it could change the rest of your life.

Chapter 15

Choking

Just as Kevin took a bite of his hot dog, his friend Peter made a goofy face and it cracked Kevin up. But it's hard to laugh and swallow food at the same time. A piece of the hot dog slipped down Kevin's throat and got stuck. He couldn't talk, he couldn't breathe—he couldn't make any sound at all.

At first Peter thought Kevin couldn't catch his breath because he was laughing so hard. But when Kevin started waving his hands and grabbing at his throat, Peter knew his friend was in trouble. He yelled for help.

A teacher rushed over to Kevin and performed a technique called the Heimlich maneuver (say: **hime**-lik mah-**noo**-ver), which caused the hot dog piece to shoot out of Kevin's mouth and land a good 6 feet away. Gross, yes. But that teacher saved Kevin's life.

What is choking?

To understand choking, you first have to understand what goes on at the back of your throat hundreds of times per day. All the food you eat and the air you breathe passes through your throat to get into your body. Food and liquid go down one pipe—the esophagus (say: ih-**sah**-fuh-gus)—to your

> About This Chapter: "Choking," April 2008, reprinted with permission from www.kidshealth.org. Copyright © 2008 The Nemours Foundation. This information was provided by KidsHealth, one of the largest resources online for medically reviewed health information written for parents, kids, and teens. For more articles like this one, visit www.KidsHealth.org, or www.TeensHealth.org.

stomach. Air goes down another pipe—the trachea (say: **tray**-kee-uh), or windpipe—to your lungs. These two pipes share an opening at the back of your throat.

So if they share an opening, how does the food know which pipe to go down? Lucky for you, your body has it all under control. A little flap of cartilage (say: **kar**-tel-ij) called the epiglottis (say: eh-pih-**glah**-tis) sits near your trachea, and every time you swallow, it springs into action. Acting like a little door, it closes off the entrance to your trachea so that food is sent down your esophagus into your stomach instead of into your lungs.

But every once in a while, especially if you are laughing while you are eating, the epiglottis doesn't close in time. A piece of food, like Kevin's hot dog, can slip down into the trachea. Most of the time, it's no big deal. Your body makes you cough and forces it back up.

You've probably experienced this. Did you ever have a sip of a drink that "went down the wrong pipe"? You probably coughed a lot and it might have been scary, but usually you're fine in just a few seconds. That's because coughing is the body's natural defense against stuff that doesn't belong in the trachea. A good cough often can clear out a piece of food—or even an object—that heads down the trachea. If a person can still breathe and talk, coughing often does the trick.

But when someone is truly choking it means the food or object is completely blocking the airway and air cannot flow into and out of the lungs. The person cannot cough the object out. They can't breathe, talk, or even make noise. They may grab at their throat or wave their arms. If the trachea remains blocked, their face may turn from bright red to blue.

The body needs oxygen to stay alive. When oxygen can't reach the lungs and the brain, a person can become unconscious, sustain brain damage, and even die within minutes. That's what makes choking such a serious emergency.

What is the Heimlich maneuver?

The Heimlich maneuver is a way to help someone who is choking. It's usually performed by another person, but there's even a way to do it on yourself, if necessary. The traditional Heimlich maneuver is to be used on adults

Choking

and children over one year old. A helper gets behind the choking person and gives a certain kind of quick squeeze in the middle of the abdomen. This squeeze sends a quick, powerful burst of air from the person's lungs upward, dislodging the problem food or object and often sending it flying out of the person's mouth.

To do it properly, it's best to learn it from a health care professional who can show you how it's done. Sometimes, kids learn the Heimlich maneuver in a health class or a first-aid class.

> ♣ **It's A Fact!!**
> Dr. Henry Heimlich, a chest surgeon, was surprised to learn how many people died from choking. But what could be done? You often can't reach in a grab the problem food or object. Surgery might work, but there isn't time. Dr. Heimlich's bright idea was to work from the inside out—to use the lungs to force out whatever the person was choking on. He introduced his idea in 1974, and it's been saving lives ever since.
>
> Source: © 2008 Nemours Foundation.

What should I do if someone is choking?

Choking is serious stuff. If you're around a person you think is choking, yell for help and have somebody call 911 right away. If you are trained to do the Heimlich maneuver, you should do it immediately. It can be a lifesaver, but it's safest when done by someone trained to perform it. If it's done the wrong way, the choking person—especially a baby or child—could be hurt.

If a choking person is unconscious and has already stopped breathing, the Heimlich needs to be performed along with cardiopulmonary resuscitation (CPR), which is also best performed by someone who knows how to do it correctly.

How can I prevent choking?

Here are four great ways to prevent choking:

1. Be extra careful when eating certain foods that are easy to choke on. They include things like: hot dogs, nuts, grapes, raw carrots, popcorn, and hard or gooey candy.

♣ It's A Fact!!
Study Warns Of Deaths
Due To The "Choking Game"

At least 82 youth have died as a result of playing what has been called "the choking game," according to a study released by the Centers for Disease Control and Prevention in *Morbidity and Mortality Weekly Report*. The choking game involves intentionally trying to choke oneself or another in an effort to obtain a brief euphoric state or "high." Death or serious injury can result if strangulation is prolonged.

Eighty-seven percent of these deaths were among males, and most fatalities occurred among those 11 years to 16 years old; the average age was 13, the report said. Choking game deaths were identified in 31 states, it said.

Signs that someone may be engaging in the choking game include the following:

- discussion of the game—including other terms used for it, such as "pass-out game" or "space monkey"
- bloodshot eyes
- marks on the neck
- severe headaches
- disorientation after spending time alone
- ropes, scarves, and belts tied to bedroom furniture or doorknobs or found knotted on the floor
- unexplained presence of things like dog leashes, choke collars, and bungee cords

The choking game is life-threatening.

Source: Excerpted from "CDC Study Warns of Deaths Due to the 'Choking Game,'" Center for Disease Control and Prevention (CDC), February 14, 2008.

Choking

2. Sit down, take small bites, and don't talk or laugh with your mouth full. Do we sound like your mom? Well, she's right. And there's more than good manners at stake. Following that advice will help prevent choking.

3. Look out for the little guys—and girls. Babies and toddlers love to put things in their mouths, so help keep them safe by picking up anything off the floor that might be dangerous to swallow—like deflated balloons, pen caps, coins, beads, and batteries. Keep toys with small parts out of reach, and never share your food or candy with a baby unless an adult says it's OK.

4. Learn the Heimlich maneuver. It's usually taught as part of any basic first-aid course—the kind that might be held by the Red Cross, the YMCA, the American Heart Association, schools, or hospitals in your community. Who knows? You could be a lifesaver someday.

Chapter 16

Drug Overdose And Alcohol Poisoning

Drug Abuse First Aid

Considerations: Many street drugs have no therapeutic benefits. Any use of these drugs is a form of drug abuse. Legitimate medications can be abused by people who take more than the recommended dose or who intentionally take them with alcohol or other drugs. Drug interactions also produce adverse effects. Therefore, it is important to let your doctor know about all the drugs you are taking.

Many drugs are addictive. Sometimes the addiction is gradual, while with others (such as cocaine), an addiction can happen after only a few doses. Someone who has become addicted to a drug will likely experience withdrawal symptoms if they suddenly stop taking it. Withdrawal is greatly assisted by professional help.

A drug dose that is large enough to be toxic is called an overdose. Prompt medical attention may save the life of someone who accidentally or deliberately takes an overdose.

Causes: An overdose of narcotics can cause sleepiness and even unconsciousness. Uppers (stimulants) produce excitement, increased rate of heartbeat,

---

About This Chapter: This chapter begins with "Drug Abuse First Aid," © 2008 A.D.A.M., Inc. Reprinted with permission. "Facts about Alcohol Poisoning," is from the National Institute on Alcohol Abuse and Alcoholism, July 11, 2007.

and rapid breathing. Downers (depressants) do just the opposite. Mind-altering drugs are called hallucinogens. They include LSD and other street drugs. Using such drugs may cause paranoia, hallucinations, aggressive behavior, or extreme social withdrawal. Cannabis-containing drugs such as marijuana may cause relaxation, impaired motor skills, and increased appetite.

Legal prescription drugs are sometimes taken in higher-than-recommended amounts to achieve a feeling other than the therapeutic effects for which they were intended. This may lead to serious side effects.

Symptoms: Drug overdose symptoms vary widely depending on the specific drug(s) used, but may include:

- Abnormal pupil size;
- Nonreactive pupils (pupils do not change size when exposed to light);
- Sweating;
- Tremors;
- Agitation;
- Convulsions;
- Staggering or unsteady gait (ataxia);
- Difficulty breathing;
- Drowsiness;
- Unconsciousness (coma);
- Hallucinations;
- Delusional or paranoid behavior;
- Violent or aggressive behavior;
- Death.

Drug withdrawal symptoms also vary widely depending on the specific drug(s) used, but may include:

- Abdominal cramping;
- Diarrhea;
- Agitation;
- Hallucinations;
- Cold sweat;
- Nausea and vomiting;
- Convulsions;
- Restlessness;
- Delusions;
- Shaking;
- Depression;
- Death.

Drug Overdose And Alcohol Poisoning

First Aid

1. Check the patient's airway, breathing, and pulse. If necessary, begin cardiopulmonary resuscitation (CPR). If the patient is unconscious but breathing, carefully place him or her in the recovery position. If the patient is conscious, loosen the clothing, keep the person warm, and provide reassurance. Try to keep the patient calm. If an overdose is suspected, try to prevent the patient from taking more drugs. Call for immediate medical assistance.

2. Treat the patient for signs of shock, if necessary. Signs include: weakness, bluish lips and fingernails, clammy skin, paleness, and decreasing alertness.

3. If the patient is having seizures, give convulsion first aid.

4. Keep monitoring the patient's vital signs (pulse, rate of breathing, blood pressure) until emergency medical help arrives.

5. If possible, try to determine which drug(s) were taken and when. Save any available pill bottles or other drug containers. Provide this information to emergency medical personnel.

DO NOT

- DO NOT jeopardize your own safety. Some drugs can cause violent and unpredictable behavior. Call for professional assistance.

- DO NOT try to reason with someone who is on drugs. Do not expect them to behave reasonably.

- DO NOT offer your opinions when giving help. You don't need to know why drugs were taken in order to give effective first aid.

> **What's It Mean?**
> Drug abuse is the misuse or overuse of any medication or drug, including alcohol.
> Source: © 2008 A.D.A.M.

When To Contact A Medical Professional

Drug emergencies are not always easy to identify. If you suspect someone has overdosed, or if you suspect someone is experiencing withdrawal, give first aid and seek medical assistance.

Try to find out what drug the person has taken. If possible, collect all drug containers and any remaining drug samples or the person's vomit for analysis.

The National Poison Control Center (1-800-222-1222) can be called from anywhere in the United States. They will give you further instructions. This is a free and confidential service. All local poison control centers in the United States use this national number. You should call if you have any questions about poisoning or poison prevention. It does not need to be an emergency. You can call for any reason, 24 hours a day, 7 days a week.

Facts About Alcohol Poisoning

Excessive drinking can be hazardous to everyone's health. Some people laugh at the behavior of others who are drunk. Some think it's even funnier when they pass out. But there is nothing funny about the aspiration of vomit leading to asphyxiation or the poisoning of the respiratory center in the brain, both of which can result in death.

Do you know about the dangers of alcohol poisoning? When should you seek professional help for a friend? Sadly enough, too many students say they wish they would have sought medical treatment for a friend. Many end up feeling responsible for alcohol-related tragedies that could have easily been prevented.

Common myths about sobering up include drinking black coffee, taking a cold bath or shower, sleeping it off, or walking it off. But these are just myths, and they don't work. The only thing that reverses the effects of alcohol is time—something you may not have if you are suffering from alcohol poisoning. And many different factors affect the level of intoxication of an individual, so it's difficult to gauge exactly how much is too much (BAC calculators).

What happens to your body when you get alcohol poisoning?

Alcohol depresses nerves that control involuntary actions such as breathing and the gag reflex (which prevents choking). A fatal dose of alcohol will eventually stop these functions.

Drug Overdose And Alcohol Poisoning

> ### ✤ It's A Fact!!
>
> Inhalant abuse, commonly called huffing, is the purposeful inhalation of chemical vapors to achieve an altered mental or physical state. Abusers inhale vapors emitted from a wide range of substances. In fact, chemical vapors used as inhalants can be found in over 1,000 common household products.
>
> Chronic inhalant abuse may result in serious and sometimes irreversible damage to the user's heart, liver, kidneys, lungs, and brain. Brain damage may result in personality changes, diminished cognitive functioning, memory impairment, and slurred speech.
>
> Death from inhalant abuse can occur after a single use or after prolonged use. Sudden sniffing death (SSD) may result within minutes of inhalant abuse from irregular heart rhythm leading to heart failure. Other causes of death include asphyxiation, aspiration, or suffocation. A user who is suffering from impaired judgment may also experience fatal injuries from motor vehicle accidents or sudden falls.
>
> Source: Excerpted from "Intelligence Brief: Huffing, The Abuse of Inhalants," U.S. Department of Justice (www.usdoj.gov), November 2001.

It is common for someone who drank excessive alcohol to vomit since alcohol is an irritant to the stomach. There is then the danger of choking on vomit, which could cause death by asphyxiation in a person who is not conscious because of intoxication.

You should also know that a person's blood alcohol concentration (BAC) can continue to rise even while he or she is passed out. Even after a person stops drinking, alcohol in the stomach and intestine continues to enter the bloodstream and circulate throughout the body. It is dangerous to assume the person will be fine by sleeping it off.

What are critical signs for alcohol poisoning?

- Mental confusion, stupor, coma, or person cannot be roused
- Vomiting
- Seizures
- Slow breathing (fewer than eight breaths per minute)

- Irregular breathing (10 seconds or more between breaths)
- Hypothermia (low body temperature), bluish skin color, paleness

What should I do if I suspect someone has alcohol poisoning?

- Know the danger signals.
- Do not wait for all symptoms to be present.
- Be aware that a person who has passed out may die.
- If there is any suspicion of an alcohol overdose, call 911 for help. Don't try to guess the level of drunkenness.

What can happen to someone with alcohol poisoning that goes untreated?

- Victim chokes on his or her own vomit
- Breathing slows, becomes irregular, or stops
- Heart beats irregularly or stops
- Hypothermia (low body temperature)
- Hypoglycemia (too little blood sugar) leads to seizures
- Untreated severe dehydration from vomiting can cause seizures, permanent brain damage, or death

> **Remember!!**
> Don't be afraid to seek medical help for a friend who has had too much to drink. Don't worry that your friend may become angry or embarrassed—remember, you cared enough to help. Always be safe, not sorry.
>
> Source: CDC, 2007.

Even if the victim lives, an alcohol overdose can lead to irreversible brain damage. Rapid binge drinking (which often happens on a bet or a dare) is especially dangerous because the victim can ingest a fatal dose before becoming unconscious.

Part Three

Motor Vehicle Safety

Chapter 17

Teen Drivers: The Facts

Motor vehicle crashes are the leading cause of death for U.S. teens, accounting for 36% of all deaths in this age group. However, research suggests that the most strict and comprehensive graduated drivers licensing programs are associated with reductions of 38% and 40% in fatal and injury crashes, respectively, of 16-year-old drivers.

- In the U.S. during 2004, 4,767 teens ages 16 to 19 died of injuries caused by motor vehicle crashes. During 2005, nearly 400,000 motor vehicle occupants in this age group sustained nonfatal injuries severe enough to require treatment in an emergency department.

- The risk of motor vehicle crashes is higher among 16 to 19-year-olds than among any other age group. In fact, per mile driven, teen drivers ages 16 to 19 are four times more likely than older drivers to crash.

- The presence of teen passengers increases the crash risk of unsupervised teen drivers; the risk increases with the number of teen passengers.

- Teens are more likely than older drivers to underestimate hazardous situations or dangerous situations or not be able to recognize hazardous situations.

About This Chapter: This chapter begins with excerpts from "Teen Drivers: Fact Sheet," Centers for Disease Control and Prevention, April 2007. Additional information from the Insurance Institute for Highway Safety, Highway Loss Data Institute is cited separately within the chapter.

- Teens are more likely than older drivers to speed and allow shorter headways (the distance from the front of one vehicle to the front of the next). The presence of male teenage passengers increases the likelihood of these risky driving behaviors among teen male drivers.

- Among male drivers between 15 and 20 years of age who were involved in fatal crashes in 2005, 38% were speeding at the time of the crash and 24% had been drinking.

- Compared with other age groups, teens have the lowest rate of seat belt use. In 2005, 10% of high school students reported they rarely or never wear seat belts when riding with someone else.

> ♣ **It's A Fact!!**
> **Groups At Risk**
> - In 2004, the motor vehicle death rate for male drivers and passengers age 16 to 19 was more than one and a half times that of their female counterparts (19.4 per 100,000 compared with 11.1 per 100,000).
> - Crash risk is particularly high during the first year that teenagers are eligible to drive.

- At all levels of blood alcohol concentration (BAC), the risk of involvement in a motor vehicle crash is greater for teens than for older drivers.

    - In 2005, 23% of drivers ages 15 to 20 who died in motor vehicle crashes had a BAC of 0.08 g/dl or higher.

    - In a national survey conducted in 2005, nearly 30% of teens reported that within the previous month, they had ridden with a driver who had been drinking alcohol. One in ten reported having driven after drinking alcohol within the same one-month period.

    - In 2005, among teen drivers who were killed in motor vehicle crashes after drinking and driving, 74% were unrestrained.

- In 2005, half of teen deaths from motor vehicle crashes occurred between 3 p.m. and midnight and 54% occurred on Friday, Saturday, or Sunday.

Beginning Drivers' Crashes Differ

Excerpted from "Beginning Teenage Drivers," © 2006 Insurance Institute for Highway Safety, Highway Loss Data Institute (www.iihs.org). Reprinted with permission.

Teen drivers have the highest crash risk of any age group. Per mile traveled, they have the highest involvement rates in crashes, from crashes involving property damage only to those that are fatal. The problem is worst among 16-year-olds, who have the most limited driving experience and an immaturity that often results in risk-taking behind the wheel. The characteristics of 16-year-olds' fatal crashes shed light on the problem (see Table 17.1.).

Table 17.1: Percentage Of Fatal Crashes By Characteristic, 2004

Characteristic	Driver Age		
	16	17–19	20–49
Driver error	78	69	55
Speeding	39	33	23
Single vehicle	52	45	39
3+ occupants	29	24	18
Drivers killed with .08+ BAC	13	25	44

Data Sources: FARS, NHTSA 2004 (Table source: Insurance Institute for Highway Safety, Highway Loss Data Institute).

- **Driver Error:** Compared with crashes of older drivers, those of 16-year-olds more often involve driver error.

- **Speeding:** 16-year-old drivers have a higher rate of crashes in which excessive speed is a factor.

- **Single-Vehicle Crashes:** More of 16-year-olds' fatal crashes involve only the teen's vehicle. Typically these are high-speed crashes in which the driver lost control.

- **Passengers:** 16 year-olds' fatal crashes are more likely to occur when other teenagers are in the car. The risk increases with every additional passenger.

- **Alcohol:** Although this is a problem among drivers of all ages, it's actually less of a problem for 16-year-olds. Typically, less than 15 percent of fatally injured 16-year-old drivers have blood alcohol concentrations of .08 grams per deciliter or greater. However, alcohol quickly becomes a problem in the later teen years.

- **Night Driving:** This is a high-risk activity for beginners. Per mile driven, the nighttime fatal crash rate for 16-year-olds is about twice as high as during the day.

- **Low Safety Belt Use:** Teenagers generally are less likely than adults to use safety belts.

Chapter 18

The Keys To Defensive Driving

If you've been out on the roads, you know that not everyone drives well. Some people speed aggressively. Others wander into another lane because they aren't paying attention. Drivers may follow too closely, make sudden turns without signaling, or weave in and out of traffic.

Aggressive drivers are known road hazards, causing one third of all traffic crashes. But inattentive driving is becoming more of a problem as people "multitask" by talking on the phone, eating, or even watching TV as they drive. We can't control the actions of other drivers. But learning defensive driving skills can help us avoid the dangers caused by other people's bad driving.

Skills That Put You In Control

Before you get behind the wheel of all that glass and steel, here are some tips to help you stay in control:

Stay Focused: There are a lot of things to think about when driving: road conditions, your speed, observing traffic laws and signals, following directions, being aware of the cars around you, checking your mirrors—the list goes on. Staying focused on driving—and only driving—is key.

> About This Chapter: "The Keys to Defensive Driving," September 2007, reprinted with permission from www.kidshealth.org. Copyright © 2007 The Nemours Foundation. This information was provided by KidsHealth, one of the largest resources online for medically reviewed health information written for parents, kids, and teens. For more articles like this one, visit www.KidsHealth.org, or www.TeensHealth.org.

Distractions, like talking on the phone or eating, make a driver less able to see potential problems and react to them. It's not just teen drivers who are at fault: People who have been driving for a while can get overconfident in their driving abilities and let their driving skills get sloppy. All drivers need to remind themselves to stay focused.

Stay Alert: Being alert (not sleepy or under the influence) allows you to react quickly to potential problems—like when the driver in the car ahead slams on the brakes at the last minute. Obviously, alcohol or drugs (including prescription and over-the-counter drugs) affect a driver's reaction time and judgment. Driving while tired has the same effect and is one of the leading causes of crashes. So rest up before your road trip.

♣ **It's A Fact!!**
The best strategy to deal with road rage is to get out of the driver's way as soon as it's safe to do so and keep lots of distance between you.

Watch Out For The Other Guy: Part of staying in control is being aware of the drivers around you and what they may suddenly do so you're less likely to be caught off guard. For example, if a car speeds past you on the highway but there's not much space between the car and a slow-moving truck in the same lane, it's a pretty sure bet the driver will try to pull into your lane directly in front of you. Anticipating what another driver may do prepares you to react.

Eight Secrets Of Super Driving

When you drive defensively, you're aware and ready for whatever happens. You are cautious, yet ready to take action and not put your fate in the hands of other drivers. According to the U.S. Department of Transportation, 90% of all crashes are attributed to driver error.

Following these defensive driving tips can help reduce your risk on the road:

1. Think safety first. Avoiding aggressive and inattentive driving tendencies yourself will put you in a stronger position to deal with other people's bad driving. Leave plenty of space between you and the car in front. Always lock your doors and wear your seatbelt to protect you from being thrown from the car in a crash.

The Keys To Defensive Driving

2. Be aware of your surroundings—pay attention. Check your mirrors frequently and scan conditions 20 to 30 seconds ahead of you. If a vehicle is showing signs of aggressive driving, slow down or pull over to avoid it. If the driver is driving so dangerously that you're worried, try to get off the roadway by turning right or taking the next exit if it's safe to do so. Also, keep an eye on pedestrians, bicyclists, and pets along the road.

3. Do not depend on other drivers. Be considerate of others but look out for yourself. Do not assume another driver is going to move out of the way or allow you to merge. Assume that drivers will run through red lights or stop signs and be prepared to react. Plan your movements anticipating the worst-case scenario.

4. Have an escape route. In all driving situations, the best way to avoid potential dangers is to position your vehicle where you have the best chance of seeing and being seen. Having an alternate path of travel is essential, so take the position of other vehicles into consideration when determining an alternate path of travel.

5. Follow the 3- to 4-second rule. Since the greatest chance of a collision is in front of you, using the 3- to 4-second rule will help you establish and maintain a safe following distance and provide adequate time for you to brake to a stop if necessary in normal traffic under good weather conditions.

6. Keep your speed down. Posted speed limits apply to ideal conditions. It's your responsibility to ensure that your speed matches conditions.

7. Separate risks. When faced with multiple risks, it's necessary to address them by separating risks. Your goal is to avoid having to deal with too many risk factors at the same time.

8. Cut out distractions. A distraction is any activity that diverts your attention from the task of driving. Driving deserves your full attention—so stay focused on the driving task.

If you're interested in taking a defensive driving course to help sharpen your driving knowledge and skills, contact your state's Department of Motor

Vehicles (DMV). All states keep a list of defensive driving courses that are approved by the state—some even offer courses online. They cost money, but some insurance companies offer insurance premium discounts for the successful completion of a course.

> ✔ **Quick Tip**
> A safe following distance depends on you speed. The faster you're going, the more space you'll need. Use the 3-second rule to make sure you're leaving enough room between you and the car ahead: Pick a fixed object on the road, like a speed limit sign. When the car in from of you passes it, slowly count three seconds. If you reach the object before you're done counting, you are following too closely. If driving conditions are bad, increase your following distance.

Chapter 19

Questions And Answers About Graduated Driver Licensing

What is graduated driver licensing?

It's a system designed to phase in young beginners to full driving privileges as they become more mature and develop their driving skills. Versions of graduated licensing are in effect in New Zealand; Victoria, Australia; and several Canadian provinces. Beginning with Florida in 1996, graduated licensing systems also have been adopted in most U.S. states.

There are three stages to a graduated system: a supervised learner's period; an intermediate license (after passing the driver test) that limits driving in high-risk situations except under supervision; and then a license with full privileges, available after completing the first two stages.

The best systems include a learner's stage, beginning at age 16 and lasting at least six months, plus restrictions on unsupervised night driving and passengers during the first six to 12 months of licensure. The nighttime driving restriction should start at 9 or 10 p.m., and no more than one passenger should be allowed with an unsupervised beginning driver anytime during the day.

> About This Chapter: "Graduated Driver Licensing," © 2006 Insurance Institute for Highway Safety, Highway Loss Data Institute (www.iihs.org). Reprinted with permission.

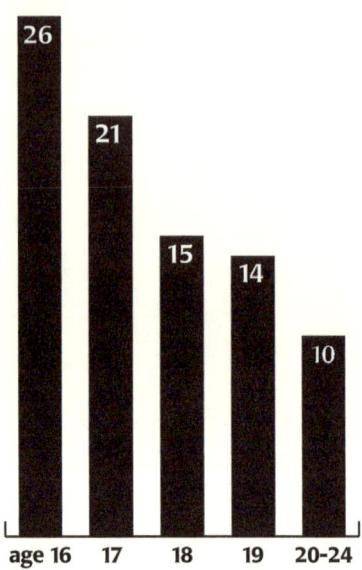

Figure 19.1. Crash Involvements Per Million Miles Driven, By Driver Age

No state law meets or exceeds all of these requirements, but most states do impose some of the core requirements. Some states add other requirements including belt use provisions, cell phone use restrictions, penalty systems so that violations result in license suspension or extension of the holding period, and driver education. For more about the licensing law in your state, or any state, go to www.iihs.org/laws/state_laws/grad_license.html.

Why target young people? Why not target all novice drivers?

Graduated licensing could apply to all first-time drivers. This is the policy in many countries. But in the United States young people make up the majority of beginning drivers, and their crash rates are particularly high. Sixteen year-olds have higher crash rates than drivers of any other age, including older teenagers.

Two factors in particular work against young drivers: inexperience behind the wheel and immaturity. Young drivers need time to develop their driving skills and the judgment to counteract their lack of on-the-road experience. Young drivers tend to overestimate their own physical and driving abilities and underestimate the dangers on the road.

The very youngest drivers are more likely to engage in risky behavior such as speeding, passing inappropriately, following other vehicles too closely, and driving without buckling their safety belts. Because of their inexperience, beginners are least able to cope with hazardous driving situations. The presence of passengers can increase the risk by distracting a beginning driver and creating peer pressure to participate in risky behavior. Teen passengers increase the crash risk for teenage drivers during the day as well as at night.

Graduated licensing doesn't attempt to modify driver behavior directly. Instead it introduces beginners to driving in a low-risk manner, protecting both them and others on the road while they learn to drive and become more mature. It should be noted that young people are subject to legal restrictions in a variety of areas that include voting, purchasing alcohol, serving in the military, and assuming financial obligations.

> ♣ **It's A Fact!!**
> **Has graduated licensing reduced crashes?**
> Yes. Sound research indicates that graduated licensing programs have had positive effects on the crash experience of young drivers in the United States and other countries, including Canada and New Zealand. In U.S. states that have adopted elements of graduated licensing, the safety benefits are evident. Almost all studies have found crash reductions from about 10 to 30 percent.

Isn't it unfair to restrict all teenagers' driving privileges? Why not just penalize the problem drivers?

We know some characteristics of younger drivers who are more likely to get into crashes, but it's impossible to identify them adequately and intervene before they crash. The licensing systems in many states impose greater and/or earlier penalties on young people for traffic violations than they do on older drivers, but most fatally injured young drivers don't have prior traffic violations or crashes on their records.

The logic of addressing all young people is that they all are beginning drivers. They all need time to develop driving skills in low-risk settings.

What are nighttime driving restrictions?

These are different from curfews, which are viewed as means to get young people off the streets and into their homes at a set time. Communities often adopt curfews to reduce criminal or mischievous behavior, but the purpose of night restrictions on driving is to protect young beginners by keeping them from driving unsupervised during the high-risk nighttime hours.

Are nighttime restrictions critical components of graduated licensing?

Yes. Four of every 10 deaths of teenagers in motor vehicles occur between 9 p.m. and 6 a.m. Studies show that nighttime driving restrictions typically are associated with crash reductions of about 40 to 60 percent during the restricted hours.

When should the nighttime restrictions begin? How early?

Almost two-thirds of all fatal nighttime crashes involving 16 year-olds occur before midnight. This is when more young people are out on the roads.

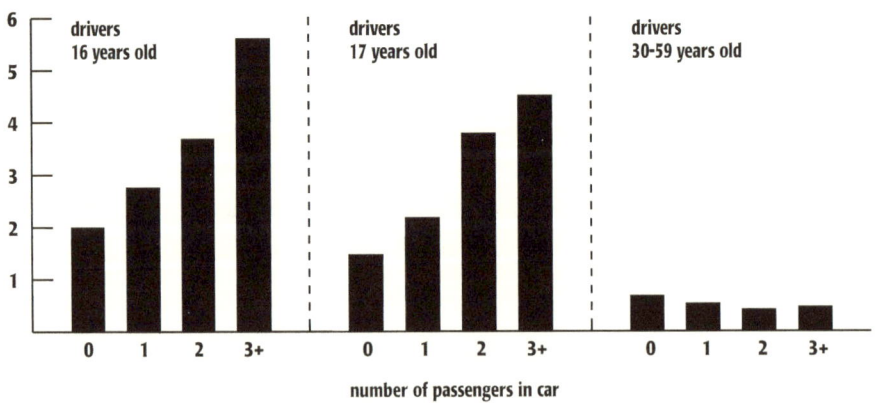

Figure 19.2. Risk When Transporting Passengers: Driver Death Rates Per 10,000 Trips, By Driver Age And Passenger Presence

Therefore, nighttime driving restrictions for young beginners should start several hours before midnight.

Are passenger restrictions important?

They're essential components of graduated licensing. Crash risk for teenage drivers increases incrementally with one, two, or three or more passengers. With three or more, fatal crash risk is about three times higher than when a beginner is driving alone.

The presence of passengers is a major contributor to the teenage death toll. Half of the crash deaths that involve 16-year-old drivers occur when the beginners are driving with teen passengers. Studies indicate that passenger restrictions can reduce this problem.

What guarantees that beginners will get more supervised driving under graduated licensing?

Requiring longer learner's permit periods (at least six months) provides more time for beginners to practice driving under the supervision of adults. Many states require parents to certify that their children have acquired a minimum amount of practice time, typically 50 hours. A survey conducted in Michigan indicates that parents are very positive about the 50-hour requirement. These parents reported an average of 75 hours of supervised driving.

Do parents support graduated licensing?

Yes, parents strongly favor it. An Insurance Institute for Highway Safety survey of parents of young drivers in California who had gone through the graduated licensing process found 95 percent of the parents in support of a six-month period of supervised driving. Ninety-four percent favored night driving restrictions, 84 percent favored restricting teenage passengers during the first six months, and 97 percent of the parents said they favor a licensing system that includes all of these components. The survey was conducted in 2000.

Parents of teens surveyed in 1996 in Connecticut, Delaware, New Jersey, and New York said they strongly support graduated licensing. Although many parents want their children to get licenses early so they no longer have to be taken to school, work, or social activities, these same parents also worry about the risks.

Are the benefits worth the costs?

States with graduated licensing report that the benefits far outweigh any costs. For example, in Oregon the administrative costs were estimated at $150,000 while the benefits were estimated at nearly $11 million. This amounts to a benefit-to-cost ratio of better than 74 to one. Maryland and California also report lifesaving and injury-reducing benefits well in excess of administrative costs.

Are teenagers allowed to drive to school, work, and their extra-curricular activities?

Yes. States can and do allow waivers so a teenager may drive during restricted times to work or to attend school activities. These exemptions don't reduce the restrictions' effectiveness because the increased crash risk at night is largely due to the combination of more difficult driving conditions and distractions caused by teenage passengers. Young people driving to work are unlikely to have teen passengers. Graduated licensing does delay full licensure, but studies indicate it doesn't significantly hinder social activities. Sixteen year-olds have largely similar lifestyles in terms of social, dating, and work patterns, whether they live in states where many, some, or few 16 year-olds are licensed. Another concern is the administrative burden on states that have to issue many waivers. Maryland examined this when it implemented a nighttime driving restriction and found it wasn't a problem.

Can driver education reduce the need for graduated licensing?

No. Driver education hasn't been shown to reduce subsequent crash rates among beginning drivers. A good education course, emphasizing on-the-road driving, can teach basic vehicle control skills. But if driver education is offered or required in a state or community, it needs to be in the framework of an effective graduated licensing system to reduce crashes. More important is that completion of driver education shouldn't reduce the time a beginner is restricted under a graduated system. No amount of driver education will take the place of actual experience behind the wheel under controlled conditions.

Chapter 20

Safety Belts And Teens

Teens have higher fatality and injury rates in motor vehicle crashes than any other age group. This may be attributable to both driving inexperience and a greater propensity for risk taking behaviors. For instance, while teens are learning the new skills needed for driving, many frequently engage in high-risk behaviors such as speeding or driving after using alcohol or other drugs, and not wearing their safety belts. Studies also have shown teens are easily distracted while driving, especially by other teen passengers. Safety belt use is one of the most effective measures to decrease injuries and deaths in a crash; unfortunately, teens are less likely to be buckled up than any other age group.

Teens Are At Risk

- Motor vehicle crashes are the leading cause of death for teens in the United States.

- In 2003, 5,240 teens were killed in passenger-vehicle crashes, and 458,000 teens were injured.

- Sixty-three percent of the fatally injured 16- to-20-year-old passenger vehicle occupants were unrestrained, compared to 55 percent for adults 21 or older.

About This Chapter: Excerpted from "Safety Belts and Older Teens—2005 Report," National Highway Traffic Safety Administration (www.nhtsa.dot.gov), March 2005.

- In 2003, the fatality rate (per 100,000 population) in motor vehicle crashes for 16- to 20-year-olds was more than twice the rate than for all other ages combined (25.7 versus 11.4 respectively).

- During 2003, a teen died in a traffic crash an average of once every hour on weekends (weekends are defined as 6 p.m. Friday through 5:59 a.m. Monday) and nearly once every two hours during the week.

> ♣ **It's A Fact!!**
> Safety belts should always be worn, even when riding in vehicles equipped with air bags. Air bags are designed to work with safety belts, not alone. In 2003, an estimated 2,488 lives were saved by air bags.

- In 2003, 34 percent (1,782) of fatally injured teens were completely or partially ejected from a passenger vehicle, compared with 27 percent of those fatally injured for all ages combined.

- Male teens are less likely to wear safety belts than female teens. In 2003, a greater number of males (7.7 percent) reported they were likely to rarely or never use safety belts when driving compared with females (2.8 percent). More males (26.4 percent) than females (23.6 percent) also reported that they had not worn their safety belts within the past week.

- A recent medical study examined motor vehicle fatality exposure rates and found the rate at which African American and Hispanic male teenagers (13 to 19 years old) are fatally injured in a motor vehicle crash is nearly twice as high as the comparable rate for white male teenagers.

- Research has shown that lap/shoulder belts, when used properly, reduce the risk of fatal injury to front-seat passenger car occupants by 45 percent and the risk of moderate to critical injury by 50 percent. For light-truck occupants, safety belts reduce the risk of fatal injury by 60 percent and moderate-to-critical injury by 65 percent.

Strong Safety Belt Laws Can Make A Difference

- There are two types of safety belt laws: primary and secondary. A primary safety belt law allows a law enforcement officer to stop a vehicle and issue a citation when the officer simply observes an unbelted driver

Safety Belts And Teens

or passenger. A secondary safety belt law means that a citation for not wearing a safety belt can only be written after the officer stops the vehicle for another infraction.

- Primary safety belt laws are much more effective in increasing safety belt use, because people are more likely to buckle up when there is the perceived risk of receiving a citation for not doing so. In 2003, the average safety belt use rate in states with primary enforcement laws was 11 percentage points higher than in states without primary enforcement laws.

- Most teens support primary enforcement safety belt laws. In 2003, a nationwide survey was conducted to determine attitudes regarding primary enforcement safety belt laws. Of those young people 16 to 20 years of age who were surveyed, 64 percent voiced their support for primary enforcement laws.

Safety Belt Enforcement Programs

- Occupant Protection Selective Traffic Enforcement Programs (sTEPs) involve periods of highly visible safety belt law enforcement combined with extensive media support. These programs are a proven method to rapidly change motorists' safety belt use behavior. Successful Occupant Protection sTEPs have been documented in Canada, Europe, and the United States.

- Highly visible enforcement of safety belt laws is a core strategy to increase safety belt use. States and communities have greater success in achieving increased safety belt use when there is strong enforcement of the law, along with effective media support. This strong enforcement of safety belt laws sends the message that the state takes safety belt use laws seriously. Ultimately, this leads to greater compliance.

- The Click It or Ticket (CIOT) model has been enormously successful in increasing safety belt use at the community, state, and regional level. This nationwide initiative, a partnership involving the National Highway Traffic Safety Administration (NHTSA), the Air Bag and Seat Belt Safety Campaign, and hundreds of law enforcement agencies, increased national belt use by four percentage points in 2003. Safety belt use increased again in 2004, reaching an all-time high of 80 percent.

- A strong graduated driver licensing (GDL) system will include education and enforcement of safety belt laws. For example, in North Carolina, the GDL law includes a provision for violations of GDL restrictions that includes safety belt infractions; a conviction extends the interim licensing period for six months from the time of the violation.

Chapter 21

What You Need To Know About Air Bags

The Air Bag System For Frontal Crashes

The air bag system consists of three basic parts—an air bag module, crash sensors, and a diagnostic unit. Some systems may also have an on/off switch, which allows the air bag to be deactivated.

The air bag module contains both an inflator unit and the lightweight fabric air bag. The driver air bag module is located in the steering wheel hub, and the passenger air bag module is located in the instrument panel. When fully inflated, the driver air bag is approximately the diameter of a large beach ball. The passenger air bag can be two to three times larger since the distance between the right-front passenger and the instrument panel is much greater than the distance between the driver and the steering wheel.

The crash sensors are located either in the front of the vehicle or in the passenger compartment. Vehicles can have one or more crash sensors. The sensors are typically activated by forces generated in significant frontal or near-frontal crashes. Sensors measure deceleration, which is the rate at which the vehicle slows down. Because of this, the vehicle speed at which the sensors activate the air bag varies with the nature of the crash. Air bags are not designed to activate during sudden braking or while driving on rough or uneven

---

About This Chapter: Excerpted from "What You Need to Know about Air Bags," National Highway Traffic Safety Administration (www.nhtsa.dot.gov), 2002.

pavement. In fact, the maximum deceleration generated in the severest braking is only a small fraction of that necessary to activate the air bag system.

The diagnostic unit monitors the readiness of the air bag system. The unit is activated when the vehicle's ignition is turned on. If the unit identifies a problem, a warning light alerts the driver to take the vehicle to an authorized service department for examination of the air bag system. Most diagnostic units contain a device, which stores enough electrical energy to deploy the air bag if the vehicle's battery is destroyed very early in a crash sequence.

When Do Air Bags Deploy?

Air bags are typically designed to deploy in frontal and near-frontal collisions, which are comparable to hitting a solid barrier at approximately eight to 14 miles per hour (mph). Roughly speaking, a 14 mph barrier collision is equivalent to striking a parked car of similar size across the full front of each vehicle at about 28 mph. This is because the parked car absorbs some of the energy of the crash, and is pushed by the striking vehicle. Unlike crash tests into barriers, real-world crashes typically occur at angles, and the crash forces usually are not evenly distributed across the front of the vehicle. Consequently, the relative speed between a striking and struck vehicle required to deploy the air bag in a real-world crash can be much higher than an equivalent barrier crash.

Because air bag sensors measure deceleration, vehicle speed and damage are not good indicators of whether or not an air bag should have deployed. Occasionally, air bags can deploy due to the vehicle's undercarriage violently striking a low object protruding above the roadway surface. Despite the lack of visible front-end damage, high deceleration forces may occur in this type of crash, resulting in the deployment of the air bag.

Most air bags are designed to automatically deploy in the event of a vehicle fire when temperatures reach 300 to 400 degrees Fahrenheit. This safety feature helps to

♣ **It's A Fact!!**
Some vehicles without rear seats, such as pick up trucks and convertibles, or with rear seats too small to accommodate rear-facing child restraints, have manual ON/OFF switches for the passenger air bag installed at the factory.

What You Need To Know About Air Bags

ensure that such temperatures do not cause an explosion of the inflator unit within the air bag module.

Front air bags are not designed to deploy in side impact, rear impact or rollover crashes. Since air bags deploy only once and deflate quickly after the initial impact, they will not be beneficial during a subsequent collision. Safety belts help reduce the risk of injury in many types of crashes. They help to properly position occupants to maximize the air bag's benefits and they help restrain occupants during the initial and any following collisions. So, it is extremely important that safety belts always be worn, even in air bag-equipped vehicles.

When A Collision Occurs

When a crash occurs, the vehicle rapidly decelerates while its structure absorbs the majority of the crash forces. Unbelted occupants continue to move forward at the vehicle's original speed until the vehicle's interior (the steering wheel, instrument panel, windshield, etc.) stops their movement. Belted occupants come to a more gradual stop by being secured to the vehicle's structure. In severe crashes, even properly belted occupants may come into contact with the vehicle's interior.

Air bags supplement the safety belt by reducing the chance that the occupant's head and upper body will strike some part of the vehicle's interior. They also help reduce the risk of serious injury by distributing crash forces more evenly across the occupant's body.

When there is a moderate to severe frontal crash that requires the frontal air bag to deploy, a signal is sent to the inflator unit within the air bag module. An igniter starts a reaction, which produces a gas to fill the air bag, making the air bag deploy through the module cover. Some air bag technologies use nitrogen gas to fill the air bag while others may use argon gas. The gases used to fill air bags are harmless.

What Happens After A Deployment?

Once an air bag deploys, deflation begins immediately as the gas escapes through vents in the fabric. Deployment is frequently accompanied by the release of dust-like particles in the vehicle's interior. Most of this dust consists

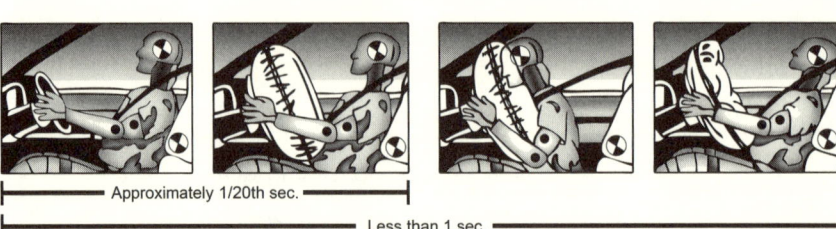

Figure 21.1. From the onset of the crash, the entire deployment and inflation process takes only about 1/20th of a second, faster than the blink of an eye. Because a vehicle changes speed so fast in a crash, air bags must inflate rapidly if they are to help reduce the risk of the occupant hitting the vehicle's interior.

of cornstarch or talcum powder, which are used to lubricate the air bag during deployment. Small amounts of sodium hydroxide may initially be present. This chemical can cause minor irritation to the eyes and open wounds; however, with exposure to air, it quickly turns into sodium bicarbonate (common baking soda). Depending on the type of air bag system, potassium chloride (a table salt substitute) may also be present.

For most people, the only effect the dust may produce is some minor irritation of the throat and eyes. Generally, minor irritations only occur when the occupant remains in the vehicle for many minutes with the windows closed and no ventilation. However, some people with asthma may develop an asthmatic attack from inhaling the dust. With the onset of symptoms, asthmatics should treat themselves as advised by their doctor, then immediately seek medical treatment.

Once deployed, the air bag cannot be reused and should be replaced by an authorized service department. Because the air bags only deploy once, do not drive the vehicle until the air bags have been replaced.

Air Bag Contact Injuries

Air bags must inflate very rapidly to be effective, and therefore come out of the steering wheel hub or instrument panel with considerable force, generally at a speed over 100 mph. Because of this initial force, contact with a deploying air bag may cause injury. These air bag contact injuries, when they occur, are typically very minor abrasions or burns.

More serious injuries are rare; however, serious or even fatal injuries can occur when someone is very close to, or in direct contact with an air bag module when the air bag deploys. Such injuries may be sustained by unconscious drivers who are slumped over the steering wheel, unrestrained or improperly restrained occupants who slide forward in the seat during pre-crash braking, and even properly restrained drivers who sit very close to the steering wheel. Never attach objects to an air bag module or place loose objects on or near an air bag module, since they can be propelled with great force by a deploying air bag, potentially causing serious injuries.

An unrestrained or improperly restrained occupant can be seriously injured or killed by a deploying air bag. The National Highway Traffic Safety Administration (NHTSA) recommends drivers sit with at least 10 inches between the center of their breastbone and the center of the steering wheel. Children 12 and under should always ride properly restrained in a rear seat. Never put a rear-facing infant restraint in the front seat of a vehicle with a front passenger air bag. A rear-facing infant restraint places an infant's head close to the air bag module, which can cause severe head injuries or death if the air bag deploys.

Air Bags, Safety Belts, And Child Safety Seats

All front seat occupants must be correctly positioned in order to optimize the benefits of a deploying air bag. The proper use of safety belts is an important part of correct positioning. Unbelted or improperly belted occupants can come into contact with the air bag module during pre-crash braking. Being near or against an air bag module when it deploys can result in serious or fatal injury.

Safety belts should always be worn with the lap belt low and snug across the hips and the shoulder belt across the chest. Shoulder belts should never be placed under the arm or behind the back. Front seat drivers and passengers should sit upright against the back of the seat. Passengers should adjust the seat as rearward as practical. Drivers should adjust the seat such that they position themselves away from the air bag module, while maintaining the ability to safely operate all vehicle controls. Moving the seat rearward, slightly reclining the seat back and/or tilting the adjustable steering wheel downward can change the driving position. Remember, NHTSA recommends there must be at least 10 inches distance between the steering wheel hub, where the air bag module is located, and the driver's breastbone.

Children are safest when properly restrained in a rear seat, whether the vehicle has an air bag or not. Infants should be restrained in rear-facing restraints until they reach 20 pounds and are at least one year of age. Never put a rear-facing infant restraint in the front seat of a vehicle with a front passenger air bag. The back of the rear-facing infant restraint rests too close to the air bag module, creating the potential for serious or fatal injuries from a deploying air bag.

After children reach 20 pounds and one year of age, they can be moved into forward-facing child restraints. When children exceed 40 pounds in weight, they should ride in belt-positioning booster seats until the vehicle safety belt fits properly, which as a rule of thumb may be until they are at least 8 years old, unless they are 4'9" tall. Most booster seats accommodate children up to 80 lbs. Always follow the child restraint and vehicle manufacturers' instructions for proper use and installation of child restraints.

New Technologies

Advanced Air Bag Technologies: Many advanced air bag technologies are being developed to tailor air bag deployment to the severity of the crash, the size and posture of the vehicle occupant, belt usage, and how close that person is to the air bag module. Many of these systems will use multi-stage inflators that deploy less forcefully in stages in moderate crashes than in very severe crashes. However, even with advanced air bag technologies, children ages 12 and under should always ride in a rear seating position in an appropriate restraint system.

Side And Rollover Air Bags: Many new vehicles are also equipped with side air bags. While there are several types of side air bags, all are designed to reduce the risk of injury

♣ **It's A Fact!!**
Pregnant women should always wear their safety belts. They should sit as far back as possible from the air bag with the lap portion of the belt correctly positioned over the hips (not the stomach) and the shoulder portion across the chest.

What You Need To Know About Air Bags

> ☞ **Remember!!**
>
> Air bags are called supplemental restraints because they are designed to work best in combination with safety belts. You should always wear your safety belt whether or not your car has an air bag. All new passenger cars, light trucks, and vans are equipped with both driver and passenger front air bags.

in moderate to severe side impact crashes. These air bags are generally located in the outboard edge of the seat back, in the door, or in the roof rail above the door. Unlike front air bags, side air bags are neither required nor regulated by NHTSA.

While side air bags are smaller than front air bags, they must deploy very rapidly. Close proximity of a child's head, neck, or chest to a side air bag may cause serious injury. Therefore, it is important never to lean up against or rest against a side air bag. Seat belts (or child restraints as appropriate) should always be worn to avoid possible injury by keeping enough distance between the occupant and the side air bag module.

Chapter 22

Tire Safety

Studies of tire safety show that maintaining proper tire pressure, observing tire and vehicle load limits (not carrying more weight in your vehicle than your tires or vehicle can safely handle), avoiding road hazards, and inspecting tires for cuts, slashes, and other irregularities are the most important things you can do to avoid tire failure, such as tread separation or blowout and flat tires. These actions, along with other care and maintenance activities, can also help in several ways:

- Improve vehicle handling
- Help protect you and others from avoidable breakdowns and accidents
- Improve fuel economy
- Increase the life of your tires

Safety First—Basic Tire Maintenance

Properly maintained tires improve the steering, stopping, traction, and load-carrying capability of your vehicle. Underinflated tires and overloaded vehicles are a major cause of tire failure. Therefore, as mentioned above, to avoid flat tires and other types of tire failure, you should maintain proper tire

---

About This Chapter: Text in this chapter is from excerpted "Tire Safety: Everything Rides on It," National Highway Traffic Safety Administration (www.nhtsa.dot.gov), October 2001.

✔ Quick Tip
What To Do If You Have A Blowout On The Highway

Having a flat tire when driving is always a problem. But experiencing a flat or blowout while traveling on an interstate highway or other high-speed roadway can present special dangers. The National Safety Council offers these tips for coping with tire trouble:

- At the first sign of tire trouble, grip the steering wheel firmly.

- Don't slam on the brakes.

- Let the car slow down gradually by taking your foot off the gas pedal.

- Work your vehicle toward the breakdown lane or, if possible, toward an exit.

- If it is necessary to change lanes, signal your intentions to drivers behind and do so smoothly and carefully, watching your mirrors and the traffic around you very closely.

- Steer as your vehicle slows down. It is better to roll the car off the roadway (when you have slowed to 30 miles per hour) and into a safe place than it is to stop in traffic and risk a rear-end or side collision from other vehicles.

- When all four wheels are off the pavement—brake lightly and cautiously until you stop.

- Turn your emergency flashers on.

- It's important to have the car well off the pavement and away from traffic before stopping, even if proceeding to a place of safety means rolling along slowly with the bad tire flapping. You can drive on a flat if you take it easy and avoid sudden moves. Don't worry about damaging the tire. It is probably ruined anyway.

- Once off the road, put out reflectorized triangles behind your vehicle to alert other drivers. Keep your emergency flashers on. If you know how to change a tire, have the equipment, and can do it safely without being near traffic, change the tire as you normally would.

Tire Safety

- Remember that being safe must take precedence over your schedule or whatever other concerns you may have. Changing a tire with traffic whizzing past can be nerve-wracking at best and dangerous at worst. Therefore, it may be best to get professional help if you have a tire problem or other breakdown on a multi-lane highway.

- Raise your hood and tie something white to the radio antenna or hang it out a window so police officers or tow truck operators will know that you need help.

- Don't stand behind or next to your vehicle. If possible, stand away from the vehicle and wait for help to arrive.

- All interstate highways and major roads are patrolled regularly. Also, some highways have special "call-for-help" phones. If you have a cell phone you can call right from the roadside. It is inadvisable to walk on a multi-lane highway. However, if you can see a source of help and are able to reach it on foot, try the direct approach by walking but keeping as far from traffic as possible.

These are the most important things to remember when dealing with a flat tire on the highway:

- Don't stop in traffic.

- Get your vehicle completely away from the roadway before attempting to change a tire.

- Tackle changing a tire only if you can do so without placing yourself in danger.

- Finally, the Council recommends that you have a qualified mechanic check your vehicle after having a flat tire to be sure there is no residual damage from the bad tire or the aftermath of the flat.

Source: "What to Do If You Have a Blowout on the Highway," © 2004 National Safety Council (www.nsc.org); reprinted with permission.

pressure, observe tire and vehicle load limits, avoid road hazards, and regularly inspect your tires.

Finding Your Vehicle's Recommended Tire Pressure And Load Limits

Tire information placards and vehicle certification labels contain information on tires and load limits. These labels indicate the vehicle manufacturer's information including the following:

- Recommended tire size
- Recommended tire inflation pressure
- Vehicle capacity weight (VCW—the maximum occupant and cargo weight a vehicle is designed to carry)
- Front and rear gross axle weight ratings (GAWR—the maximum weight the axle systems are designed to carry)

Both placards and certification labels are permanently attached to the vehicle door edge, door post, glove-box door, or inside of the trunk lid. You can also find the recommended tire pressure and load limit for your vehicle in the vehicle owner's manual.

Understanding Tire Pressure And Load Limits

Tire inflation pressure is the level of air in the tire that provides it with load-carrying capacity and affects the overall performance of the vehicle. The tire inflation pressure is a number that indicates the amount of air pressure—measured in pounds per square inch (psi)—a tire requires to be properly inflated. (You will also find this number on the vehicle information placard expressed in kilopascals (kPa), which is the metric measure used internationally.)

Manufacturers of passenger vehicles and light trucks determine this number based on the vehicle's design load limit, that is, the greatest amount of weight a vehicle can safely carry and the vehicle's tire size. The proper tire pressure for your vehicle is referred to as the "recommended cold inflation pressure."

Tire Safety

> ♣ **It's A Fact!!**
>
> **Checking Tire Pressure**
>
> It is important to check your vehicle's tire pressure at least once a month for the following reasons:
>
> - Most tires may naturally lose air over time.
> - Tires can lose air suddenly if you drive over a pothole or other object or if you strike the curb when parking.
> - With radial tires, it is usually not possible to determine underinflation by visual inspection.
>
> For convenience, purchase a tire pressure gauge to keep in your vehicle. Gauges can be purchased at tire dealerships, auto supply stores, and other retail outlets.
>
> The recommended tire inflation pressure that vehicle manufacturers provide reflects the proper psi when a tire is cold. The term cold does not relate to the outside temperature. Rather, a cold tire is one that has not been driven on for at least three hours. When you drive, your tires get warmer, causing the air pressure within them to increase. Therefore, to get an accurate tire pressure reading, you must measure tire pressure when the tires are cold or compensate for the extra pressure in warm tires.
>
> Source: NHTSA, 2001.

Because tires are designed to be used on more than one type of vehicle, tire manufacturers list the "maximum permissible inflation pressure" on the tire sidewall. This number is the greatest amount of air pressure that should ever be put in the tire under normal driving conditions.

Steps For Maintaining Proper Tire Pressure

- Step 1: Locate the recommended tire pressure on the vehicle's tire information placard, certification label, or in the owner's manual.
- Step 2: Record the tire pressure of all tires.

- Step 3: If the tire pressure is too high in any of the tires, slowly release air by gently pressing on the tire valve stem with the edge of your tire gauge until you get to the correct pressure.
- Step 4: If the tire pressure is too low, note the difference between the measured tire pressure and the correct tire pressure. These "missing" pounds of pressure are what you will need to add.
- Step 5: At a service station, add the missing pounds of air pressure to each tire that is underinflated.
- Step 6: Check all the tires to make sure they have the same air pressure (except in cases in which the front and rear tires are supposed to have different amounts of pressure).

If you have been driving your vehicle and think that a tire is underinflated, fill it to the recommended cold inflation pressure indicated on your vehicle's tire information placard or certification label. While your tire may still be

♣ **It's A Fact!!**
Tire Repair

The proper repair of a punctured tire requires a plug for the hole and a patch for the area inside the tire that surrounds the puncture hole. Punctures through the tread can be repaired if they are not too large, but punctures to the sidewall should not be repaired. Tires must be removed from the rim to be properly inspected before being plugged and patched.

Source: NHTSA, 2001.

Tire Safety

slightly underinflated due to the extra pounds of pressure in the warm tire, it is safer to drive with air pressure that is slightly lower than the vehicle manufacturer's recommended cold inflation pressure than to drive with a significantly underinflated tire. Since this is a temporary fix, don't forget to recheck and adjust the tire's pressure when you can obtain a cold reading.

Tire Size

To maintain tire safety, purchase new tires that are the same size as the vehicle's original tires or another size recommended by the manufacturer. Look at the tire information placard, the owner's manual, or the sidewall of the tire you are replacing to find this information. If you have any doubt about the correct size to choose, consult with the tire dealer.

Tire Tread

The tire tread provides the gripping action and traction that prevent your vehicle from slipping or sliding, especially when the road is wet or icy. In general, tires are not safe and should be replaced when the tread is worn down to 1/16 of an inch. Tires have built-in tread wear indicators that let you know when it is time to replace your tires. These indicators are raised sections spaced intermittently in the bottom of the tread grooves. When they appear "even" with the outside of the tread, it is time to replace your tires. Another method for checking tread depth is to place a penny in the tread with Lincoln's head upside down and facing you. If you can see the top of Lincoln's head, you are ready for new tires.

Tire Balance And Wheel Alignment

To avoid vibration or shaking of the vehicle when a tire rotates, the tire must be properly balanced. This balance is achieved by positioning weights on the wheel to counterbalance heavy spots on the wheel-and-tire assembly. A wheel alignment adjusts the angles of the wheels so that they are positioned correctly relative to the vehicle's frame. This adjustment maximizes the life of your tires and prevents your car from veering to the right or left when driving on a straight, level road. These adjustments require special equipment and should be performed by a qualified technician.

Tire Rotation

Rotating tires from front to back and from side to side can reduce irregular wear (for vehicles that have tires that are all the same size). Look in your owner's manual for information on how frequently the tires on your vehicle should be rotated and the best pattern for rotation.

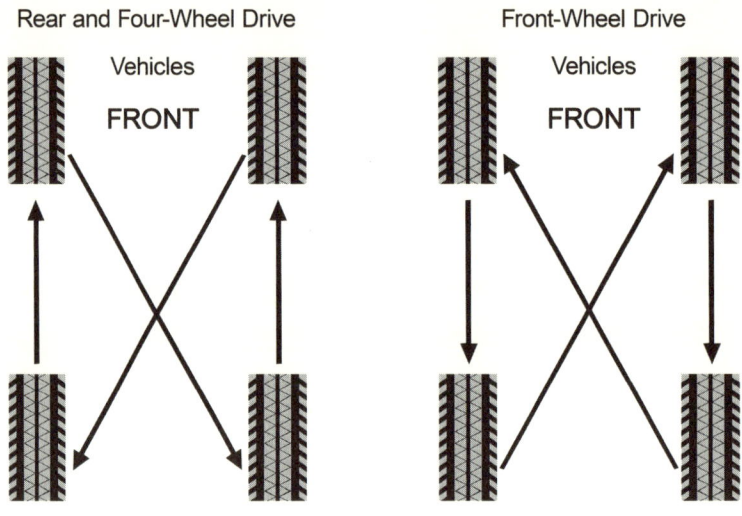

Figure 22.1. A Tire Rotation Example: For maximum mileage, rotate your tires every 5,000 miles. Follow correct rotation patterns.

Chapter 23

Headlights And Safer Night Driving

If bright lights have been bothering you more lately when you drive at night, you're not alone. The comment above, like hundreds of other complaints received recently by the government and AAA clubs across the country, indicates that glare from headlights has flared into a bigger problem than ever.

But you don't need to continue to suffer. With the right strategies, the right driving techniques, and the right equipment, you can fight back at nighttime glare.

New Lights, Old Problems

Drivers have been complaining about glare ever since electric headlights began replacing oil lamps on automobiles more than 85 years ago. So what's the big deal now? Why does glare seem to have grown worse? The answer involves technology, automotive design, and demographics.

Extra Lights: Many vehicles now sport fog lamps or other auxiliary lights in front. Ideally, fog lamps cast a low, broad beam to reduce "back-scatter" from the vehicle's headlights when water droplets hang in the air. They're intended to improve a driver's ability to see in foggy, misty, or hazy conditions. However, when they're aimed improperly or used on clear nights, they can annoy other drivers.

About This chapter: "Blinded by the Light?" © 2002 AAA Foundation for Traffic Safety (www.aaafoundation.org). Reprinted with permission.

High-Tech Lights: Introduced in Europe in 1996, high-intensity discharge (HID) lights are showing up on more cars in the United States, especially upscale models. Unlike conventional bulbs, HID headlights don't have filaments. Instead, they use a high-voltage electrical arc to ionize xenon gas and make it glow. HIDs emit twice the light of halogen headlamps, but also produce a blue-white light. Other headlights look yellow by comparison.

Whether you love HIDs or hate them depends on which side of the light you're on. Drivers with HIDs swear by them, while other drivers swear at them. Many motorists who are faced with HID lights find the amount of light and its blue-white quality blinding.

Higher Lights: After years of steady growth, sales of SUVs and light trucks have surpassed sales of passenger cars. Many of these larger vehicles—especially the four-wheel-drive variety—ride higher than cars. As a result their headlights ride higher, too. Although no headlights can exceed the 54-inch height limit set by federal safety standards, the lights on SUVs typically measure about 33 inches—almost 9 inches higher than headlights on passenger cars. It's no wonder car drivers often complain that the lights on big 4X4s shine directly in their eyes.

Off-Kilter Lights: Headlights pointed as little as one degree too high can make a huge difference to oncoming drivers. Misaimed beams also don't cast as much light on the road, where it counts. Unfortunately, studies show that almost half the vehicles in states that require regular inspections had at least one improperly aimed headlight. Vehicles more than five years old are twice as likely to have off-kilter headlights as newer ones.

Your Eyes: Like beauty, glare is often in the eye of the beholder. Middle-aged and older drivers are more sensitive to glare than younger drivers because their eyes take longer to adjust to changing light levels. As the population ages, the number of older drivers will continue to rise—and complaints about glare will rise, too. Lighter-colored eyes are more sensitive, which means the lighter your eyes are the more glare will bother you. Certain other conditions, such as having had vision-correction surgery that affects the corneas, may also increase your sensitivity to glare.

✔ Quick Tip
Do-It-Yourself Headlight Alignment

You'll Need

- A level
- A spacious parking area near a flat, light-colored wall
- A tape measure
- Masking tape

- Park so that both the left and right headlights are precisely 25 feet from the wall.

- Using your tape measure, find the exact middle of both the windshield and rear window and mark them with strips of tape, creating vertical centerlines front and rear.

- Standing behind the car, now sight along those centerlines, as if you were lining up sights on a rifle in a carnival shooting gallery. When centerlines are aligned you can locate the headlight centerline on the wall. Mark this with another strip of tape.

- Now measure the distance between headlight lenses, center to center. Divide the headlight-to-headlight distance in half and measure that distance to the right of the centerline on the wall. Mark it with a vertical strip of tape. Do same to the left side.

- Finally, measure the distance from the ground to the center of each headlight lens; mark that distance on the wall with a horizontal strip of tape. You should now have two crosses on the wall, with centers that correspond exactly to the center of each headlight lens.

- Turn your headlights on low beam. The left edge of the bright spots on the wall should just touch the vertical bars of the crosses in the lower-right quadrants. The top edge should just touch the horizontal bars. On some cars, you can adjust the headlight aim yourself by turning small set screws at the top and sides of each lamp.

If you cannot do it yourself, a mechanic can adjust your headlights at a garage or dealership. Aligning your headlights does not substitute for any required state inspections.

Prepare To Fight Glare

Even before you hit the road, prepare yourself and your vehicle for combating the bright lights ahead.

Clean Your Headlights: When you squeegee your windshield at the gas station, be sure to clean your headlights, too. Even a thin layer of road grime on the lenses can block up to 90 percent of the light and severely restrict your ability to see at night.

Clean lenses are even more important if you have HID headlights. Dirt diffuses the light from HIDs and causes glare that can temporarily blind other drivers, so headlight-cleaning systems are standard equipment on many cars with HIDs. Using the headlight cleaners regularly becomes a matter of "enlightened" self-interest for you; when you reduce glare for oncoming drivers you improve your own safety as well. After all, everybody shares the same road.

Keep All Glass Clear—Really Clear: Streaks, smudges, and road grime on your windows catch and refract light. This includes the inside of your windshield. Chemicals from the plastic in your car's interior slowly build up on the glass, until pretty soon you're looking at the windshield, not through it. Scratched eyeglasses or contact lenses also make glare worse. For maximum glare prevention, keep every surface between your eyes and the road as clear as possible—including both sides of your windshield and your eyeglasses. Clean the windows (inside and out!) at least once a month to get rid of haze—more often if you smoke in the car.

While you're at it, clean your wiper blades with a paper towel dipped in windshield washer fluid. This removes grime and oxidized rubber from the edge of the blade and helps prevent streaking. If streaks persist, you need new blade refills. (These are available at any auto parts store or discount chain.)

Have chips or cracks in the windshield repaired, pronto. Often a trained glass repair technician can fill small damaged areas with special resin—a fast, inexpensive process that not only improves visibility but also prevents the crack or chip from growing and requiring a windshield replacement.

Aim Your Headlights Correctly: If you live in a state that requires regular safety inspections, ask the technician to check and correct the aim of your

Headlights And Safer Night Driving

headlights. If your state doesn't require such an inspection, take your vehicle to a dealer or other properly equipped repair shop at least once a year for a headlight checkup. Your properly aligned headlights will help you see the road better, and will help other drivers avoid glare.

Adjust Both Outside Mirrors: Properly aligned mirrors not only reduce blind spots, they also reduce glare from vehicles behind you.

AAA recommends the following method: While sitting in the driver's seat, lean to the left and tilt your head until it rests against the window. From that position, adjust the driver's side mirror so you can just see the left rear fender. Next, while sitting in the driver's seat, lean to the right and tilt your head until it's in the center of the vehicle. From that position, adjust the passenger-side mirror so that the right rear fender is just visible.

Now when cars pass you, you'll notice that your mirrors don't direct the brightest part of the headlights into your eyes. You'll also notice that the arrangement reduces blind spots and makes it easier to spot vehicles to the side and rear.

Have Your Vision Checked Regularly: The American Optometric Association recommends that everyone under age 40 have a thorough eye exam at least every three years; drivers 41 to 60, every two years; and drivers over age 60, every year. Age makes eyes more sensitive to glare, but certain medical conditions, such as encroaching cataracts, will increase the problem. If the problem is detected early, your eye care professional can recommend effective treatment.

Behind-The-Wheel Tips

A few simple but surprisingly effective techniques will help you fight glare:

Avert Your Eyes: When oncoming vehicles shine light directly into your eyes, look down and to the right. Turn your gaze to the white line on the right side of the road, or to where pavement meets the shoulder, until the vehicle goes by. You can still see the vehicles around you with your peripheral vision, but the glare won't bother you as much because you are not using the most light-sensitive part of your eyes.

Use The Mirror's "Night" Setting: All cars have "day/night" interior mirrors to reduce reflected glare from vehicles directly behind you. You can change the mirror to its "night" setting by flipping the small lever at the bottom of the mirror. This changes the angle of the reflective surface and appears to dim the mirror. Lights will still show up in the glass, but they're much less bright and not so bothersome.

Use Your Lights Courteously: If your car has fog lamps, don't use them if there is no fog. In fog, use only your low-beam headlights; high beams reduce your own ability to see and may temporarily blind other drivers. Avoid using your high beams when you see oncoming vehicles or when you drive in urban areas.

Take Frequent Breaks: If you're driving at night for a long time, stop often to reduce fatigue and give your eyes a chance to recover. Take a short nap, or at least a brisk walk and some caffeine to help you stay alert.

Extra Glare Protection

OK, you prepped your car completely for night driving. You've had your eyes checked by a professional. And you've tried the behind-the-wheel techniques above. But glare still bothers you. Don't give up. Try these strategies:

Anti-Reflective Eyeglass Coating: Many eye care professionals strongly recommend glasses with an anti-reflective (AR) coating. This ultrathin film, made from zircon and silicon, reduces internal reflections in the lenses. Unlike sunglasses or self-darkening lenses, which block some light, AR-coated glasses actually transmit more light—about eight percent more. This improves vision at night and helps distinguish fine details during the day. Highway patrol troopers have reported better night and day vision and reduced nighttime glare with AR-coated lenses. These lenses may help you, too.

Self-Dimming Mirrors: Many upscale cars now offer self-dimming mirrors that reduce glare but allow you to maintain excellent rearward visibility. As the glare becomes brighter, the mirrors become darker; as the glare diminishes, the mirrors lighten up. These mirrors are available from some dealers and automobile parts stores. If you're particularly sensitive to reflected glare,

Headlights And Safer Night Driving

consider getting self-dimming mirrors, either as replacements for your current mirrors or as equipment on your next car.

If All Else Fails: Drivers with vision problems may find that even these techniques don't help. In that case, think about driving less at night, or restricting your travel to routes that have good overhead roadway lighting and clear, well-maintained pavement markings.

♣ **It's A Fact!!**
Think Twice Before...

Using "night-driving" glasses. Some marketers offer specially tinted glasses (usually yellow) that supposedly block the wavelengths of light responsible for most troublesome glare. Unfortunately, no matter what their tint, these glasses also reduce the amount of light that reaches your eyes, and you need light to see. While these glasses may reduce glare, they also reduce your night vision overall—hardly a safe bargain.

Wearing sunglasses at night. Eye care professionals warn against wearing sunglasses at night or indoors. They not only restrict your night vision but eventually, as your eyes get used to them, they become inadequate for daytime protection.

Installing "blue-light specials" on your car. Status-seekers who envy the blue-white HID headlights on upscale cars often fall for the fake HIDs offered by some manufacturers as replacements. Even though they may have "xenon" or "blue" in their names, they're often just ordinary halogen headlights that have been given a blue tint. Because of the added coloring they may actually provide less light than regular bulbs. If you must replace your headlights, don't buy cheap, imitation HIDs; consider using the lights recommended by your vehicle's manufacturer.

Chapter 24

Bad-Weather Driving Tips

Your parents and other adults may talk about the great privilege of driving. However, to you driving may just mean freedom to finally go where you want when you want.

But at times, factors beyond your control can affect driving conditions and even compromise your safety on the road. These include: rain, wind, snow, ice, bright sun, fog, and everyone's favorite—hail—just to name a few. So what should you do if you find yourself stuck driving in bad weather?

Braving The Elements

The term "joy ride" does not apply when it's pouring and the wind is gusting. The best strategy for driving in bad weather is to avoid it.

But if going out is necessary or you get caught in bad conditions once you're already out, follow these safe driving tips:

- Make sure your headlights are on.
- Increase your following distance—if you're going slowly because of bad weather, is there really a point to being only two feet behind the car in front of you?

> About This Chapter: "Bad-Weather Driving," September 2007, reprinted with permission from www.kidshealth.org. Copyright © 2007 The Nemours Foundation. This information was provided by KidsHealth, one of the largest resources online for medically reviewed health information written for parents, kids, and teens. For more articles like this one, visit www.KidsHealth.org, or www.TeensHealth.org.

- Slow down. Braking takes longer on slippery roads—the slower you go, the easier it will be for you to stop.
- Make sure your car is prepared for the conditions (check your battery, antifreeze, windshield wiper fluid, windshield wipers, headlights, tires).
- Use caution near intersections. Never assume that because you have the green light or the right of way that the intersection will be clear—always scan ahead to spot potential hazards.
- Stay in one lane as much as possible—avoid unnecessary lane changes (don't go zipping in and out of traffic and passing people).
- Keep two hands on the wheel and two eyes on the road at all times.

BRRRRRRRaving The Snow And Ice

Driving a car is never "easy," but this is especially true in wintry weather. To hone your skills, ask someone with winter driving experience to take you to a vacant parking lot where you can practice driving, turning, and stopping in the snow.

If you must travel, keep your car gassed up so that the fuel lines don't freeze. Clear snow completely off the car, remembering to sweep the taillights and headlights. Watch out for slow-moving vehicles like snowplows and sand trucks, and try not to get too close—the last thing you need in a snowstorm is a windshield full of sand. Also try to avoid passing these vehicles.

> ✔ **Quick Tip**
> **All Hail Storms**
> Perhaps one of the oddest things to deal with in a car is a hailstorm which often comes out of nowhere. Windshield wipers are not made for golf ball-sized chunks of ice, nor is the body of your car. If you can, slowly pull under the cover of a bridge or garage to avoid further damage to your car. If you aren't near anything, pull over and onto the shoulder, put on your flashers, and wait for the flying ice to stop.

Bad-Weather Driving Tips

Put together a car emergency kit that contains:

- an ice scraper and a snow brush;
- a bag of sand, salt or cat litter (for traction if you get stuck in snow);
- warning flares or triangles;
- blankets;
- gloves or mittens;
- a flashlight and batteries;
- a first-aid kit;
- booster cables;
- nonperishable snack foods;
- a candle and matches;
- a cup in case you need to melt snow for water.

> ♣ **It's A Fact!!**
> **News Flash On Flash Flooding**
> The term "flash flood" is on the news all the time, but it probably never concerned you before you were driving. Flash floods are caused by a lot of rain in a little time. They can strike without warning—before proper signs can be posted and roads can be closed. If you see standing water, of any depth, avoid it and find a higher route.

If you get stranded, stay with your vehicle and call for assistance. Run the heater occasionally to keep warm, but avoid carbon monoxide poisoning by making sure your tailpipe isn't stuffed or blocked with snow or other debris.

Rainy Roads

Roads are dirty places. Between tires stirring up gravel and engines dripping oil and other fluids, a lot of oily and slick substances build up on roads. That's why roads are at their slickest almost immediately after it starts raining. The water brings those oils to the surface, making it sneaky-slick.

If you get caught in a slick situation and your car starts gliding or hydroplaning, don't panic or slam on the brakes. Take your foot off the gas and gradually press the brakes, making sure not to turn the steering wheel. To avoid hydroplaning:

- make sure your tires aren't bald;
- easy does it around turns;
- if you can, go around puddles.

> ✔ **Quick Tip**
>
> **Driving In A Wind Tunnel**
>
> Although it's a gorgeous sunny day, that doesn't mean driving conditions are perfect. Wind can cause even the heavies of cars to sway or veer abruptly. Take extra care if you're in a high car, like an SUV, minivan, or truck, because these are more susceptible to heavy winds. Also be aware that open spaces and bridges are extra-windy. If your car starts to blow, keep both hands on the wheel and hold steady.

Many states require drivers to have their headlights on if it's raining. Also, be aware of thunderstorm warnings. If a thunderstorm starts while you're driving and visibility is poor, pull over and wait it out. Don't run the risk of being struck by lightning—stay in your car and pull as far off the road as safely possible.

Scorching Sun And Fuzzy Fog

One of the most vital parts of driving is visibility. Both bright sun and soupy fog can cause limited visibility. To combat that pesky fireball in the sky, always have UV sunglasses somewhere in the car. Also, to reduce bad glare, pop down the visor.

Fog can be a little trickier to handle than bright sunlight. Fog can reduce visibility to less than ¼ mile. Fog can also trick you into thinking you're going slower than you really are, so keep the speed down. When you can't see far ahead, it's hard to see brake lights or traffic signs until you're almost upon them. And just because you can't see doesn't mean that your high beams will improve visibility. In fact, high beams reduce visibility in fog. If your car has fog lamps, though, use them.

No matter what's causing the bad driving conditions, just remember: Don't venture out if you don't have to.

Chapter 25

Drowsy Driving

What Is Drowsy Driving?

Sleepiness and driving is a dangerous combination. Most people are aware of the dangers of drinking and driving but don't realize that drowsy driving can be just as fatal. Like alcohol, sleepiness slows reaction time, decreases awareness, impairs judgment, and increases your risk of crashing.

It's nearly impossible to determine with certainty the cause of a fatal crash where drowsy driving is suspected. However, there are a number of clues at a crash scene that tell investigators that the person fell asleep at the wheel. For example, drowsy driving accidents usually involve only one vehicle where the driver is alone and the injuries tend to be serious or fatal. Also, skid marks or evidence of other evasive maneuvers are usually absent from the drowsy driving crash scene.

Unlike alcohol-related crashes, no blood, breath, or other objective test for sleepiness behind the wheel currently exists that investigators could give to a driver at the scene of a crash. This makes police training in identifying drowsiness as a crash factor very difficult.

About This Chapter: This chapter includes "What Is Drowsy Driving?" "Who Is At Risk?" "Warning Signs," and "Countermeasures," © 2007 National Sleep Foundation (www.nsf.org); reprinted with permission.

Definitions of drowsy driving or driver fatigue rely on how the concept of "fatigue" is defined. Fatigue is a general term commonly used to describe the experience of being "sleepy," "tired," "drowsy," or "exhausted." While all of these terms have different meanings in research and clinical settings, they tend to be used interchangeably in the traffic safety and transportation fields.

There are many underlying causes of sleepiness, fatigue, and drowsy driving, including sleep loss from restriction or too little sleep, interruption, or fragmented sleep; chronic sleep debt; circadian factors associated with driving patterns or work schedules; undiagnosed or untreated sleep disorders; time spent on a task; the use of sedating medications; and the consumption of alcohol when already tired. These factors have cumulative effects and a combination of any of these can greatly increase one's risk for a fatigue-related crash.

Sleepiness or fatigue causes the following:

- Impaired reaction time, judgment, and vision
- Problems with information processing and short-term memory
- Decreased performance, vigilance, and motivation
- Increased moodiness and aggressive behaviors

In addition to the dangers of driving under the influence of fatigue, several states are considering legislation that would allow police to charge drowsy drivers with criminal negligence if they injure or kill someone while driving if they have not had adequate sleep.

Who's At Risk?

In general, since all humans require sleep on a daily basis, any driver can succumb to fatigue or be at higher risk for experiencing a decrease of alertness or microsleep when they have not obtained adequate sleep (both in quality and quantity).

There are many underlying causes of sleepiness, drowsiness, fatigue, and drowsy driving. They include sleep loss from restriction, interruption, or fragmentation; chronic sleep debt; circadian factors associated with driving patterns or work schedules; time on task; the use of sedating medications; and

Drowsy Driving

the consumption of alcohol when already tired. These factors have cumulative effects and a combination of any of these increases crash risk greatly.

The risk of having a crash due to drowsy driving is not uniformly distributed across the population. This is due to two factors. First, crashes tend to occur at times in keeping with one's circadian rhythms when sleepiness is most pronounced, for example, during the night and in the mid-afternoon. Thus individuals who drive at night are much more likely to have fall-asleep crashes. Second, people who are excessively sleepy either because of lifestyle factors or because of an untreated sleep disorder are more likely to have crashes related to excessive daytime sleepiness. Research has identified young males, shift workers, commercial drivers, and people with untreated sleep disorders or with short-term or chronic sleep deprivation as being at increased risk for having a fall-asleep crash.

Specific At-Risk Groups

- Young people—especially males under age 26
- Shift workers and people with long work hours—working the night shift increases your risk by nearly six times; rotating-shift workers and people working more than 60 hours a week need to be particularly careful
- Commercial drivers—especially long-haul drivers—at least 15% of all heavy truck crashes involve fatigue
- People with undiagnosed or untreated disorders—people with untreated obstructive sleep apnea have been shown to have up to a seven times increased risk of falling asleep at the wheel
- Business travelers—who spend many hours driving or may be jet lagged

Warning Signs

Your eyelids droop and your head starts to nod. Yawning becomes almost constant and your vision seems blurry. You blink hard, focus your eyes, and suddenly realize that you've veered onto the shoulder or into oncoming traffic for a moment and quickly straighten the wheel. This time you were lucky; next time you could become the latest victim of the tragedy of drowsy driving.

> ✔ **Quick Tip**
>
> ### Are You At Risk?
>
> Before you drive, consider whether you are:
>
> - sleep-deprived or fatigued (six hours of sleep or less triples your risk);
> - suffering from sleep loss (insomnia), poor quality sleep, or a sleep debt;
> - driving long distances without proper rest breaks;
> - driving through the night, mid-afternoon, or when you would normally be asleep;
> - taking sedating medications (antidepressants, cold tablets, antihistamines);
> - working more than 60 hours a week (increases your risk by 40%);
> - working more than one job and your main job involves shift work;
> - drinking even small amounts of alcohol;
> - driving alone or on a long, rural, dark, or boring road.
>
> Source: From "Who Is At Risk?" © 2007 National Sleep Foundation.

According to the National Sleep Foundation's Sleep in America poll, 60% of Americans have driven while feeling sleepy and 37% admit to actually having fallen asleep at the wheel in the past year. However, many people cannot tell if or when they are about to fall asleep. And if sleepiness comes on while driving, many say to themselves, "I can handle this, I'll be fine." Yet they're putting themselves and others in danger. What they really need is a nap or a good night's sleep.

Here are some signs that should tell a driver to stop and rest:

- Difficulty focusing, frequent blinking, or heavy eyelids
- Daydreaming; wandering/disconnected thoughts
- Trouble remembering the last few miles driven; missing exits or traffic signs
- Yawning repeatedly or rubbing your eyes
- Trouble keeping your head up
- Drifting from your lane, tailgating, or hitting a shoulder rumble strip
- Feeling restless and irritable

Countermeasures

Before "Hitting The Road"

- Get adequate sleep—most adults need seven to nine hours to maintain proper alertness during the day.
- Schedule proper breaks—about every 100 miles or two hours during long trips.
- Arrange for a travel companion—someone to talk with and share the driving.
- Avoid alcohol and sedating medications—check your labels or ask your doctor.

Countermeasures To Prevent A Fall-Asleep Crash While Driving

- Watch for the warning signs of fatigue.
- Stop driving—pull off at the next exit, rest area, or find a place to sleep for the night.
- Take a nap—find a safe place to take a 15- to 20-minute nap.
- Consume caffeine—the equivalent of two cups of coffee can increase alertness for several hours.
- Try consuming caffeine before taking a short nap to get the benefits of both.

♣ **It's A Fact!!**
Caffeine—Does It Help?

Caffeine promotes short-term alertness. It takes about 30 minutes for caffeine to begin working so the best thing to do is pull over for a coffee or other caffeinated beverage, take a short nap, and then get back on the road. Keep in mind that caffeine won't have much of an effect on people who consume it regularly.

Source: From "Countermeasures," © 2007 National Sleep Foundation.

Chapter 26

Young Drivers And Alcohol

Young drivers are over-represented in alcohol related driving accidents. Although drinking, binge drinking, and alcohol related crashes are dropping among young people, specific actions are recommended to further reduce traffic accidents involving alcohol.

The Problem

Young people are over-represented in driving accidents involving alcohol. In a recent year, people aged 16 to 24 were involved in 28 percent of all alcohol-related driving accidents, although they make up only 14% of the U.S. population. Young people are also over-represented in drinking driver injuries and deaths. Even when their blood alcohol contents (BACs) are not high, young drinkers are involved in driving accidents at higher rates than older drivers with similar BACs.

Teens and other young people may be over-represented in drunk driving accidents because, in part, they tend to:

- be relatively inexperienced drivers;
- be relatively inexperienced consumers of alcohol;

About This Chapter: "Young Drivers and Alcohol," © 2007 David J. Hanson, PhD. Reprinted with permission.

- be more likely to use illegal drugs;
- have a false sense of invincibility and immortality.

The Good News

Fortunately, driving accidents have been declining among young people, just as they have among the general population. And deaths associated with young drinking drivers (those 16 to 24 years of age) are down dramatically, having dropped 47% in a recent 15-year period.

In contrast to popular belief, drinking among young people is dropping and has been doing so for many years. For example, statistics demonstrate that within a period of about 20 years, the proportion of American high school seniors who:

- have ever consumed alcohol is down 13%;
- have consumed alcohol within the previous year is down 15%;
- have consumed alcohol within previous 30 days is down 27%;
- have recently consumed alcohol daily is down 67%;
- have "binged" (consumed 5 or more drinks on an occasion within previous two weeks) is down 24%.

Drinking Among Young People In General Continues To Drop

The proportion of youths aged 12 through 17 who consumed any alcohol within the previous month has plummeted from 50% in 1979 to 19% in 1998, according to the federal government's National Household Survey on Drug Abuse. Thus, the proportion of young drinkers has dropped in 1998, the most recent year for which statistics are available, from one in two to under one in five in 1979.

The proportion of both junior and senior high school students who have consumed any alcohol during the year has dropped again for the third year in a row, according to the PRIDE Survey, a nation-wide study of 138,079 students. The Survey is designated by federal law as an official measure of substance use by teen-agers in the United States.

> **♣ It's A Fact!!**
> **Honestly!**
>
> Unfortunately, exaggerating the extent of drinking problems on campus creates a self-fulfilling prophesy. When young people go off to college falsely believe that "everybody is drinking heavily," then they tend to conform in order to fit in as a college student. Thus, those who exaggerate the problem of alcohol abuse actually contribute to the problem and make it worse.
>
> When students find out that most others don't drink as much as they incorrectly believed, they feel empowered to drink less. So, honest accuracy rather than dishonest exaggeration is the most effective way to reduce alcohol abuse and the problems often associated with it.

Drinking Among College Students Continues To Drop

The proportion of American college students who abstain from alcohol has increased 16% between 1989–1991 and 1995–1997, according to the federally funded CORE Institute at Southern Illinois University.

The proportion of first year college students who drink beer has fallen dramatically and recently reached the lowest point in over 30 years. Similar drops have been documented in collegiate wine and spirits consumption over the past decade by UCLA's Higher Education Research Institute.

So-called bingeing is not only down among high school seniors but is also down among college students, and has been declining for a number of years.

"Binge" drinking dropped significantly among college students in the United States in the four-year period between a recent study by Dr. Henry Wechsler of Harvard and his earlier study. He also found that the proportion of college students who abstain from alcohol jumped nearly 22% that short period of time.

College student "binge" drinking recently reached the lowest level in the nearly twenty years that that the University of Michigan's Institute for Social

Research (ISR) has conducted its surveys for the National Institute on Drug Abuse. The proportion of college students who drink has also reached a record all-time low according to ISR research.

College Students Drink Less Than People Think

College students simply don't drink as much as everyone seems to think they do, according to researchers using Breathalyzers at the University of North Carolina at Chapel Hill. Even on the traditional party nights of Thursday, Friday, and Saturday, 66% of the students returned home with absolutely no blood alcohol content; two of every three had not a trace of alcohol in their systems even on party nights.

"I'm not surprised by these results," said Rob Foss, manager of Alcohol Studies for the UNC Highway Safety Research Center, which conducted the study with funding from the National Highway Traffic Safety Administration and the North Carolina Governor's Highway Safety Program. "Other Breathalyzer studies we have done with drivers and recreational boaters show similar results—less drinking than is generally believed. We have substantial misperceptions about alcohol use in this country."

The Task

While drinking abuse, including drunk driving, is down dramatically among young people, much remains to be done. Too many young people are still needlessly killed or injured as a result of drinking and driving.

We Need To Reduce Drinking And Driving

- Social pressure is very effective in reducing drunk driving.
    - Never condone or approve of intoxication. Intoxicated behavior is dangerous and never amusing.
    - Don't ever let your friends drive after drinking. Take away their keys, have them stay the night, have them ride home with someone else, or do whatever else is necessary—but don't let them drive!
- Designated driver programs save lives

Young Drivers And Alcohol 183

- Volunteer to be a designated driver. It could save your life and the lives of your friends.
- It's important to realize that inexperienced drinkers become intoxicated with much less alcohol than do experienced drinkers and are much more likely to have traffic accidents after consuming small amounts alcohol. Even a single drink dramatically increases the chances that a teen-aged driver will have a driving accident.

• Graduated penalties for driving with higher BACs could save lives.

- Faster speeders get higher speeding fines and higher blood alcohol contents (BACs) should get higher penalties. Drivers with blood alcohol contents of .20 are hundreds of times more dangerous than those with only .02 and should receive much higher penalties.

We Need To Reduce Drugging And Driving

For safe driving, never use illegal drugs. Illicit drugs are involved in a large proportion of driving accidents, injuries, and deaths. Marijuana and other drugs reduce coordination, reaction time, and other abilities required to drive safely. In the case of marijuana, this impairment lasts as long as 24 hours after smoking just one joint.

As many as nearly 40% of injured drivers have tested positive for marijuana and the proportion is probably much higher for young drivers. Police almost never test for illegal drug use and many accidents blamed on alcohol are actually caused by illicit drugs.

We Need To Improve Driver Education

Prospective drivers should be taught adequate information on alcohol and driving and they should be tested on this material on their driver's exams. In too many states, the subject is given only brief mention and seven states do not include any information or testing on it in the process of obtaining a driver's license.

We Need To Increase Safe Driving

Don't drive when fatigued. The dangers posed when fatigued are similar to those when intoxicated. Drunk or fatigued drivers both have slowed reactions and impaired judgment. Drivers who drift off cause about 72,500 injuries and deaths every year according to federal estimates. Drowsy driving is a major problem for young people, especially males 18 to 25, because they tend not to get enough sleep.

Avoid driving late on weekends. Alcohol-related driving accidents are much more likely to occur at night and on weekends.

♣ **It's A Fact!!**

Don't use a car phone, apply make-up, comb your hair, or eat while driving. Drivers using car phones have about the same chance of having an accident as driving drunk! And hands-free cell phones are just as dangerous to use while driving.

Chapter 27

Drugged Driving

What is drugged driving?

"Have one [drink] for the road" was, until recently, a commonly used phrase in American culture. It has only been within the past 20 years that as a nation, we have begun to recognize the dangers associated with drunk driving. Through a multipronged and concerted effort involving many stakeholders, including educators, media, legislators, law enforcement, and community organizations, such as Mothers Against Drunk Driving (MADD), the nation has seen a decline in the numbers of people killed or injured due to drunk driving. It is now time that we recognize and address the similar dangers that can occur with drugged driving.

In 12 states (Arizona, Georgia, Indiana, Illinois, Iowa, Michigan, Minnesota, Nevada, Pennsylvania, Rhode Island, Utah, and Wisconsin), it is illegal to operate a motor vehicle with any detectable level of a prohibited drug, or its metabolites, in the driver's blood. Other state laws define "drugged driving" as driving when a drug "renders the driver incapable of driving safely," or "causes the driver to be impaired."

In reality, the principal concern regarding drugged driving is that driving under the influence of any drug that acts on the brain could impair one's

---

About This Chapter: Excerpted from "NIDA InfoFacts: Drugged Driving," National Institute on Drug Abuse, October 2007. The complete text, including references, is available online at http://www.nida.nih.gov/Infofacts/driving.html.

motor skills, reaction time, and judgment. Drugged driving is a public health concern because it puts not only the driver at risk, but passengers and others who share the road.

How many people take drugs and drive?

The National Highway Traffic Safety Administration (NHTSA) reports that 17,000 people were killed in alcohol-related crashes in 2006. Studies also have found that drugs are used by 10 to 22 percent of drivers involved in crashes, often in combination with alcohol.

According to the 2006 National Survey on Drug Use and Health (NSDUH), an estimated 9.5 million people age 12 and older reported driving under the influence of illicit drugs during the year prior to being surveyed. This corresponds to 4.2 percent of the population aged 12 or older, similar to the rate in 2005 (4.3 percent), but lower than the rate in 2002 (4.7 percent). In 2006, the rate was highest among young adults aged 18 to 25 (13.0 percent). In addition:

- In 2006, an estimated 13.3 percent of persons aged 12 or older drove under the influence of an illicit drug or alcohol at least once in the past year. This percentage has dropped since 2005, when it was 14.1 percent. The 2006 estimate corresponds to 31.7 million persons.

- Driving under the influence of an illicit drug or alcohol was associated with age. In 2006, an estimated 7.3 percent of 16 year olds drove under the influence. This percentage steadily increased with age to reach a peak of 31.8 percent among 22 year olds. Beyond the age of 22 these rates showed a general decline with increasing age.

- Also in 2006, among persons aged 12 or older males were nearly twice as likely as females (17.6 vs. 9.3 percent) to drive under the influence of an illicit drug or alcohol in the past year.

In recent years, drugs other than alcohol that act on the brain have increasingly been recognized as hazards to road traffic safety. Research examining these drugs indicates that marijuana is the most prevalent illegal drug detected in impaired drivers, fatally injured drivers, and motor vehicle crash victims. A variety of other drugs, such as benzodiazepines, cocaine, opiates,

Drugged Driving

and amphetamines, have also been reported in fatal and nonfatal motor vehicle crashes.

A number of studies have examined illicit drug use in drivers involved in motor vehicle crashes, reckless driving, or in fatal accidents. For example:

- A recent study found that 34 percent of drivers admitted to a Maryland trauma center tested positive for drugs only, while 16 percent tested positive for alcohol only; 50 percent of those under 18 tested positive for alcohol and/or drugs. While it is interesting that more people in this study tested positive for drugs-only compared to alcohol-only, it should be noted that this represents one geographic location, so findings cannot be generalized. In fact, many studies among similar populations have found higher prevalence rates of alcohol compared with drug use.

- Studies conducted in a number of localities have found that approximately 4–14 percent of drivers who sustained injury or death in traffic accidents tested positive for delta-9-tetrahydrocannabinol (THC), the active ingredient in marijuana.

- In a large study of almost 3,400 fatally injured drivers from three Australian states (Victoria, New South Wales, and Western Australia) between 1990 and 1999, drugs other than alcohol were present in 26.7 percent of the cases. These included cannabis (13.5 percent), opioids (4.9 percent), stimulants (4.1 percent), benzodiazepines (4.1 percent), and other psychotropic drugs (2.7 percent). Almost 10 percent of the cases involved both alcohol and drugs.

Why is drugged driving hazardous?

Drugs act on the brain and can alter perception, cognition, attention, balance, coordination, reaction time, and other faculties required for safe driving. The effects of specific drugs of abuse differ depending on their mechanisms of action, the amount consumed, the history of the user, and other factors.

Marijuana: THC affects areas of the brain that control the body's movements, balance, coordination, memory, and judgment abilities, as well as

> ♣ **It's A Fact!!**
> **Teens And Drugged Driving**
>
> - According to NHTSA, vehicle accidents are the leading cause of death among those aged 15 to 20. It is generally accepted that because teens are the least experienced drivers as a group, they have a higher risk of being involved in an accident compared with more experienced drivers. When this lack of experience is combined with the use of marijuana or other substances that impact cognitive and motor abilities, the results can be tragic.
>
> - National Institute on Drug Abuse (NIDA)'s Monitoring the Future survey indicated that, in 2006, more than 10 percent of high school seniors admitted to driving under the influence of marijuana in the two weeks prior to the survey.
>
> - The 2004 State of Maryland Adolescent Survey indicates that 13.5 percent of the State's licensed adolescent drivers reported driving under the influence of marijuana on three or more occasions.

sensations. Because these effects are multifaceted, more research is required to understand marijuana's impact on the ability of drivers to react to complex and unpredictable situations.

Prescription Drugs: Many medications (for example, benzodiazepines and opiate analgesics) act on systems in the brain that could impair driving ability. In fact, many prescription drugs come with warnings against the operation of machinery—including motor vehicles—for a specified period of time after use. When prescription drugs are taken without medical supervision (that is, when abused), impaired driving and other harmful reactions can also result.

> ☞ **Remember!!**
> Drugged driving is a dangerous activity that puts us all at risk.

Chapter 28

Inattentive And Aggressive Driving

Teen Unsafe Driving Behaviors

Motor vehicle crashes are the leading cause of death for 15- to 20-year-olds, causing roughly one-third of all deaths for this age group. Teenagers are over represented in traffic crashes both as drivers and as passengers. On the basis of miles driven, teenagers are involved in three times as many fatal crashes as all other drivers. The high crash-involvement rate for this age group is caused primarily by their lack of maturity and driving experience coupled with their overconfidence and risk-taking behaviors. High-risk behaviors include failure to wear safety belts, speeding, and driving while impaired (by alcohol or other drugs), and drowsy or distracted driving. This age group is particularly susceptible to distractions caused by other passengers in the vehicle, electronic devices, and music.

- A larger percentage of fatal crashes involving teenage drivers are single-vehicle crashes compared to those involving other drivers. In this type of fatal crash, the vehicle usually leaves the road and overturns or hits a roadside object such as a tree or pole.

About This Chapter: This chapter includes excerpts from the following publications of the National Highway Traffic Safety Administration: "Teen Unsafe Driving Behaviors: Focus Group Final Report," September 2006, "NHTSA Policy and FAQs on Cellular Phone Use While Driving," "Define Aggressive Driving," 2000, "Are You An Aggressive Driver?" October 2000, and "Stop Speeding Before It Stops You," 2007.

- In general, fewer teens wear their safety belts compared to other drivers.
- A larger proportion of teen fatal crashes involve speeding, or going too fast for road conditions, compared to other drivers.
- More teen fatal crashes occur when passengers, usually other teenagers, are in the car than do crashes involving other drivers. Two out of three teens who die as passengers are in vehicles driven by other teenagers.

Findings By Selected Program Areas

Although the purpose of this project was to obtain information to assist in the design of messages for teen drivers, so much information was learned about highway safety programs, it seemed worthwhile to pick out some of these insights and present them in the paragraphs below. Please be advised that these comments reflect the insights and beliefs of the focus and affinity group participants. These statements do not necessarily reflect the views of the Department of Transportation.

- Teens "feel the need to speed," to borrow a popular quote from the movie *Top Gun*. They do not consider driving 5 or 10 miles above the speed limit to be dangerous. Rather, it is perceived as just keeping up with traffic, which many were advised to do in Driver's Ed. Focus groups indicate they may need facts to counter the effects of popular films like *The Fast and the Furious*.
- Many young male participants complain about other drivers who fail to signal their lane changes or who drive in the left lane, because they make it difficult to swerve from lane to lane at very high speeds. The young male participants believe that they are totally focused on the road ahead and can anticipate every action, thereby minimizing the risk of collision. They do not see their driving as being aggressive, just highly skilled. Steps must be taken to educate these young men about reaction times and the laws of physics.
- Focus groups suggest that teen participants do not seem to see the relationship between the numerous things that distract them in their cars and their high rate of minor fender-bender type crashes. A high percentage of the crashes reported by the teens involved rear-ending a car that had stopped while the teen driver was looking away from the

Inattentive And Aggressive Driving

road. If teens cannot be dissuaded from multitasking while driving, perhaps they should be encouraged to increase their following distance to provide a longer buffer zone.

- Focus groups indicate that teen drivers need to be empowered to impose some rules on their passengers. They all recognize the risks caused by lots of passengers: tickling them, covering their eyes, shouting out directions, and egging them on to do stupid things. However, they do not seem to have the confidence or strategies for keeping their passengers under control.

- Cell phones are not perceived as a serious risk by most teen participants, yet they complain about other drivers who do stupid things while talking on their cell phones. They do not seem to connect the many close calls that they have had while driving when using their cell phones. They need to be reminded what conditions make it too risky to answer or make a call.

- Focus groups suggest that music plays a huge part in a teenager's life, especially when they are driving. The prospect of a long or short trip with no music is almost intolerable. Yet teen participants acknowledge that adjusting the radio or switching CDs causes them to look away from the road and that crashes can occur in those milliseconds of inattention.

Cellular Phone Use While Driving

The primary responsibility of the driver is to operate a motor vehicle safely. The task of driving requires full attention and focus. Cell phone use can distract drivers from this task, risking harm to themselves and others. Therefore, the safest course of action is to refrain from using a cell phone while driving.

Does cell phone use while driving cause traffic crashes?

Research shows that driving while using a cell phone can pose a serious cognitive distraction and degrade driver performance. The data are insufficient to quantify crashes caused by cell phone use specifically, but NHTSA estimates that driver distraction from all sources contributes to 25 percent of all police-reported traffic crashes.

♣ It's A Fact!!

Driver inattention is the leading factor in most crashes and near-crashes, according to a landmark research report released in 2006 by the National Highway Traffic Safety Administration (NHTSA) and the Virginia Tech Transportation Institute (VTTI). Nearly 80 percent of crashes and 65 percent of near-crashes involved some form of driver inattention within three seconds before the event. Primary causes of driver inattention are distracting activities, such as cell phone use, and drowsiness.

The most common distraction for drivers is the use of cell phones. However, the number of crashes and near-crashes attributable to dialing is nearly identical to the number associated with talking or listening. Dialing is more dangerous but occurs less often than talking or listening.

Reaching for a moving object increased the risk of a crash or near-crash by 9 times; looking at an external object by 3.7 times; reading by 3 times; applying makeup by 3 times; dialing a hand-held device (typically a cell phone) by almost 3 times; and talking or listening on a hand-held device by 1.3 times.

Drivers who engage frequently in distracting activities are more likely to be involved in an inattention-related crash or near-crash. However, drivers are often unable to predict when it is safe to look away from the road to multi-task because the situation can change abruptly leaving the driver no time to react even when looking away from the forward roadway for only a brief time.

Source: Excerpted from "NHTSA, Virginia Tech Transportation Institute Release Findings of Breakthrough Research on Real-World Driver Behavior, Distraction and Crash Factors," National Highway Traffic Safety Administration, April 2006.

Inattentive And Aggressive Driving

Is it safe to use hands-free (headset, speakerphone, or other device) cell phones while driving?

The available research indicates that whether it is a hands-free or hand-held cell phone, the cognitive distraction is significant enough to degrade a driver's performance. This can cause a driver to miss key visual and audio cues needed to avoid a crash.

In an emergency should I use my cell phone while driving?

As a general rule, drivers should make every effort to move to a safe place off of the road before using a cell phone. However, in emergency situations a driver must use their judgment regarding the urgency of the situation and the necessity to use a cell phone while driving.

What do the studies say about the relative risk of cell phone use when compared to other tasks like eating or drinking?

The current research does not provide a definitive answer as to which behavior is riskier. In a controlled study, comparing eating and operating a voice-activated cell phone to continuously operating a CD player, it was found that the CD player operation was more distracting than the other activities. In a test track study conducted by NHTSA, the results showed that manual dialing was about as distracting as grooming/eating, but less distracting than reading or changing CDs. It is also important to keep in mind that some activities are carried out more frequently and for longer periods of time and may result in greater risk.

Aggressive Driving

Define Aggressive Driving

The National Highway Traffic Safety Administration (NHTSA) defines aggressive driving as, "when individuals commit a combination of moving traffic offenses so as to endanger other persons or property." Some other communities define aggressive driving as "the operation of a motor vehicle involving three or more moving violations as part of a single continuous sequence of driving acts, which is likely to endanger any person or property."

Road rage differs from aggressive driving. It is a criminal offense and is "an assault with a motor vehicle or other dangerous weapon by the operator or passenger(s) of one motor vehicle on the operator or passenger(s) of another motor vehicle or is caused by an incident that occurred on a roadway."

Some behaviors typically associated with aggressive driving include: exceeding the posted speed limit, following too closely, erratic or unsafe lane changes, improperly signaling lane changes, and failure to obey traffic control devices (stop signs, yield signs, traffic signals, railroad grade cross signals, etc.). NHTSA calls the act of red light running one of the most dangerous forms of aggressive driving.

Are You An Aggressive Driver?

- **Do you express frustration?** Taking out your frustrations on your fellow motorists can lead to violence or a crash.

- **Do you fail to pay attention when driving?** Reading, eating, drinking or talking on the phone, can be a major cause of roadway crashes.

✔ **Quick Tip**
When Confronted With Aggressive Drivers

- **Get out of the way:** First and foremost make every attempt to get out of their way.

- **Put your pride aside:** Do not challenge them by speeding up or attempting to hold-your-own in your travel lane.

- **Avoid eye contact:** Eye contact can sometimes enrage an aggressive driver.

- **Gestures:** Ignore gestures and refuse to return them.

- **Report serious aggressive driving:** You or a passenger may call the police. But, if you use a cell phone, pull over to a safe location.

From "Are You An Aggressive Driver?" NHTSA, October 2000.

Inattentive And Aggressive Driving

> ### ❧ What's It Mean?
>
> Speeding is usually defined as driving in excess of the posted speed limit or driving too fast for conditions and can have dangerous consequences including:
>
> - Reducing a driver's ability to negotiate curves or maneuver around obstacles in the roadway;
> - Extending the distance traveled before a vehicle can stop;
> - Increasing the distance a vehicle travels while the driver reacts to a hazard;
> - Increasing the risk of crashes and injuries because other vehicles and pedestrians may not be able to judge distance accurately.
>
> Source: NHTSA, 2005.

- **Do you tailgate?** This is a major cause of crashes that can result in serious deaths or injuries.
- **Do you make frequent lane changes?** If you whip in and out of lanes to advance ahead, you can be a danger to other motorists.
- **Do you run red lights?** Do not enter an intersection on a yellow light. Remember flashing red lights should be treated as a stop sign.
- **Do you speed?** Going faster than the posted speed limit, being a "road racer" and going too fast for conditions are some examples of speeding.

Stop Speeding Before It Stops You

- According to the National Highway Traffic Safety Administration (NHTSA), more than 13,000 lives were lost across America in speeding-related traffic crashes in 2005.
- Crash data since 1995 shows a continuous increase in the number of deaths and injuries attributed to speed. Despite gains in vehicle safety and passenger protection, thousands of Americans still die each year in speed-related crashes.

- Among drivers involved in fatal crashes, young males are the most likely to have been found speeding. In 2005, 38 percent of the males age 15–20 who were involved in fatal crashes were speeding at the time of the crash.

- Speeding motorcyclists are also over represented in crashes. In 2005, 34 percent of all motorcyclists involved in fatal crashes were speeding at the time, compared with 22 percent for passenger car drivers, 18 percent for light-truck drivers and 7 percent for large-truck drivers.

- In 2005, 25 percent of speeding drivers under age 21 who were involved in fatal crashes had a blood alcohol concentration (BAC) of .08 or higher. In contrast, only 11 percent of non-speeding drivers under age 21 involved in fatal crashes had a BAC of .08 or higher.

☞ **Remember!!**

Drivers need to remember that there is a reason for posted speed limits. The roadways are a dangerous place and the speed limits are designed to protect everyone—drivers, passengers, pedestrians—everyone.

Source: NHTSA, 2005.

Chapter 29

What To Do After A Car Accident

Alex was excited to finally get his license. He was looking forward to going to the movies and to visit friends without needing someone to take him.

A couple weeks later, Alex was headed to his friend Matt's house. Two blocks from Matt's, Alex waited at a stop sign when he felt a sudden jolt. Someone had rear-ended his car. Alex started panicking—and his first thought was "What do I do now?"

Car Crashes

In 2005 alone, there were more than 6.1 million police-reported traffic crashes in the United States. Combine those with the number of incidents that aren't reported to the police and it adds up to a lot of collisions.

Although you do your best to drive responsibly and defensively, it's still smart to know what to do just in case you end up in an accident. Crashes can be very scary, but here are some tips if one happens to you:

Take some deep breaths to get calm. After a crash, a person may feel a wide range of emotions—shock, guilt, fear, nervousness, or anger—all of

> About This Chapter: "What to Do after a Car Accident," September 2007, reprinted with permission from www.kidshealth.org. Copyright © 2007 The Nemours Foundation. This information was provided by KidsHealth, one of the largest resources online for medically reviewed health information written for parents, kids, and teens. For more articles like this one, visit www.KidsHealth.org, or www.TeensHealth.org.

which are normal. But take a few deep breaths or count to 10 to calm down. The calmer you are, the better prepared you will be to handle the situation. This is the time to take stock of the accident and try to make a judgment about whether it was a serious one.

Keep yourself and others safe. If you can't get out of your car—or it's not safe to try—keep your seat belt fastened, turn on your hazard lights, then call 911 if possible and wait for help to arrive. If you can drive your car and are in an unsafe spot or are blocking traffic, find a safe and legal place to park your car (like the shoulder of a highway or a parking lot). In some states it's illegal to move your car from the scene of an accident, though. Ask your driver's educations instructor what the law is in your state.

If the car accident seems to be minor, turn off your car and grab your emergency kit. If it's safe to get out and move around your car, set up orange cones, warning triangles, or emergency flares around the accident site.

Reporting The Accident

Check on everyone involved in the crash to see if they have any injuries. This includes making sure you don't have any serious injuries. Be extremely

---

♣ It's A Fact!!
What's in an emergency kit?

- Cell phone
- Pen and paper
- Card with information about medical allergies or conditions that may require special attention if there are serious injuries
- White cloth
- List of names and numbers for rescue personnel to contact
- A set of cones, retroreflective warning triangles, or self-lighting emergency flares
- First-aid kit
- Insurance and registration cards

What To Do After A Car Accident

cautious—not all injuries can be seen. If you or anyone involved in the accident isn't feeling 100%, you should call 911 or any other number your state uses to request emergency assistance on roadways. Be ready to give the dispatcher the following information:

- Who? The dispatcher will ask for your name and phone numbers in case the authorities need to get more information from you later.

- What? Tell the dispatcher as much as you can about the emergency—for instance, whether there is a fire, traffic hazard, medical emergency, etc.

- Where? Let the dispatcher know exactly where the emergency is taking place. Give the city, road name, road number, mile markings, direction of travel, traffic signs, and anything else you can think of to help them know how to find you.

Make sure you stay on the line until the dispatcher says it's OK to hang up.

Sometimes, you can get the police to report to the scene of the accident even if there are no injuries, especially if you tell them you need someone to mediate—in other words, to help you figure out what happened and who's at fault. But in certain areas, as long as both vehicles can be safely driven away, police officers won't come to the scene unless someone is hurt. If the police do not come to the scene, make sure you file a vehicle accident report at a police station or Department of Motor Vehicles (DMV).

Take Down Driver Information

If you are feeling up to it, ask to see the driver's license of the other drivers involved in the crash so that you can take down their license numbers. Also get their name, address, phone number, insurance company, insurance policy number, and license plate number. If the driver doesn't own the car involved, be sure to get owner's info as well.

Take Notes On The Accident

If the car accident is minor and you feel that you can describe it, try to do so. Detailed notes and photos of the scene may help the court and insurance agencies decide who is responsible for the accident. Get a good description of the cars involved—year, make, model, and color. If your phone has a camera, use that or another camera to take photos of the accident scene—including the cars and any damage, the roads, any traffic signs, and the direction each car was coming from.

If you feel well enough, try to draw a diagram of the exact crash site and mark where each car was, what direction the car was coming from, and what lane it was in. Also, write down the date, time, and weather conditions. If there were any witnesses, try to get their names and contact info so that they can help clear up matters if one of the other drivers isn't completely honest about what really happened.

Remember, you can only do these things if you think the accident was a minor one (for instance, if the airbag did not inflate). Even if you think the accident was your fault, it may not be. That's why insurance companies say that you should not admit fault or accept blame at the scene.

The Aftermath

While the crash itself might be upsetting, dealing with the aftermath can be too. In the hours or days following an accident, some people may still be shaken up. They may be beating themselves up over what happened—especially if they feel the accident was avoidable. Sometimes, people close to those who were involved in the accident (like families and best friends) can experience some emotional problems too. These feelings are all normal. Once some time passes, the car is repaired, and the insurance companies are dealt with, most accidents become mere afterthoughts.

In some cases, though, these feelings can get stronger or last for longer periods of time, keeping a person from living a normal life. Post-traumatic stress disorder (PTSD) can occur when a person has experienced a devastating event that injured or threatened to injure someone. Signs of PTSD may show up immediately following the accident, or weeks or even months after.

Not everyone who experiences stress after a trauma has PTSD. But here are some symptoms to look out for:

- Avoiding emotions or any reminders of the incident
- Constant feelings of anxiousness, crankiness, or anger

What To Do After A Car Accident

- Avoiding medical tests or procedures
- Constantly reliving the incident in one's mind
- Nightmares or trouble sleeping

If you notice any of these symptoms after you've been in a car accident, try talking through the experience with friends or relatives you trust. Discuss what happened, and what you thought, felt, and did during the accident and in the days after. Try to get back into your everyday activities, even if they make you uneasy. If these things don't help, ask your parent or guardian to help you check in with your doctor.

Other Road Problems

Most car accidents aren't as serious as a collision. Plenty of people have minor incidents—like running over the mailbox while backing out of the driveway. Somewhere between hitting mailboxes and hitting other cars are common problems like blowouts and breakdowns.

Flat Tires

Getting a flat tire while you're driving can be jarring—literally. There are some things you can do to prevent this—make sure your tires aren't too old and check the tire pressure at the gas station at least once a month. If you do find yourself in a blowout situation, though, here are a few suggestions from the National Safety Council to get you through it unharmed:

- Safely bring your car out of traffic and stop. Once you realize you have tire trouble, firmly hold the steering wheel. Don't slam on the brakes—instead, gently take your foot off the gas pedal and let the car slow down. Steer your car toward the breakdown lane or exit (if you are on the highway) or a parking lot (if you are on a smaller road). It's important to get out of the way of traffic, even if you have to drive (very cautiously) on the flat tire to do it. When your car is in a safe place, brake gently until you come to a complete stop.
- Set up your breakdown site. Once safely off the road and out of the line of traffic, turn on your emergency flashers. Take out your warning signs (cones, triangles, or flares) and place them behind your car so

that others realize that your car is disabled. If you know how to change your tire and can do it safely without getting too close to traffic, do it.

- Get help if you need it. Raise the hood of your car and hang a white T-shirt or rag out the window or off the radio antenna so that police officers and tow truck operators will know you need help. Don't try to flag down other vehicles. Use a cell phone, a highway emergency phone, or a pay phone to call for assistance. Only walk along a multi-lane highway if you can see a phone or someone who can help you nearby.

- Don't walk in or get near traffic. Does this really need further explaining?

- After it's done: Take your car to the shop so a mechanic can make sure there's no long-term damage to your car.

Breakdowns

If your car breaks down, safely bring the car to a stop and out of the line of traffic. Set up your breakdown site out of traffic. A major difference between flat tires and breakdowns is that it's less likely that you will be able to fix a car that has broken down. That's why it's wise to signal that you need help by properly displaying the white cloth and calling for roadside assistance or the police.

If you manage to get your car safely out of traffic, wait inside with the doors locked. If someone stops and offers to help you, just open the window slightly and tell them you've already called for help. Again, only walk along a multi-lane highway if you can see help nearby, and stay as far away from traffic as possible.

Chapter 30

Motorcycle Safety

Cycle Safety

You already know how much fun riding a motorcycle can be. There's nothing quite like the exhilaration of cruising the open road and the challenge of controlling a spirited motorcycle. But motorcycling also can be dangerous. The latest vehicle mile travel data show motorcyclists are about 27 times as likely as passenger car occupants to die in a motor vehicle traffic crash and six times as likely to be injured. Safe motorcycling takes balance, coordination, and good judgment. Here are some ways to ensure that you'll be around to enjoy riding your motorcycle for many years to come.

Before You Take To The Road

Make Sure You Are Properly Licensed

Driving a car and riding a motorcycle require different skills and knowledge. Although motorcycle-licensing regulations vary, all states require a motorcycle license endorsement to supplement your automobile driver's license. To receive the proper endorsement in most states, you'll need to pass written and on-cycle skills tests administered by your state's licensing agency.

About This Chapter: This chapter includes information from "Cruisin' without Bruisin'," National Highway Traffic Safety Administration (NHTSA), DOT HS 808 096, revised September 2004; and excerpts from "Traffic Safety Facts: Motorcycles," NHTSA's National Center for Statistics and Analysis, 2006.

Some states require you to take a state-sponsored rider education course. Others waive the on-cycle skills test if you've already taken and passed a state-approved course. Either way, completing a motorcycle rider education course is a good way to ensure you have the correct instruction and experience it takes to ride a motorcycle. For the motorcycle rider-training course nearest you, call the Motorcycle Safety Foundation at (800) 446-9227.

Practice Operating Your Motorcycle

Given the fact that motorcycles vary in handling and responsiveness, be sure to take the time to get accustomed to the feel of a new or unfamiliar motorcycle by riding it in a controlled area. Once you feel comfortable with your bike, you can take it into traffic. Make sure you know how to handle your motorcycle in a variety of conditions (for example, inclement weather or encountering hazards such as slick roads, potholes, and road debris). If you plan to carry cargo or a passenger, be prepared to make adjustments to the tires, suspension, and placement of the load.

> ♣ **It's A Fact!!**
> Per vehicle mile traveled, motorcyclists are about 37 times more likely than passenger car occupants to die in a traffic crash.
>
> Source: NHTSA, 2006.

Be Sure Your Motorcycle Is Safe

Before every ride, you should check the tire pressure and tread depth, hand and foot brakes, headlights and signal indicators, and fluid levels. You should also check under the motorcycle for signs of oil or gas leaks. If you're carrying cargo, you should secure and balance the load on the cycle; and adjust the suspension and tire pressure to accommodate the extra weight.

If you're carrying a passenger, he or she should mount the motorcycle only after the engine has started; should sit as far forward as possible, directly behind you; and should keep both feet on the foot rests at all times, even when the motorcycle is stopped. Remind your passenger to keep his or her legs and feet away from the muffler. Tell your passenger to hold on firmly to your waist, hips, or belt; keep movement to a minimum; and lean at the same time and in the same direction as you do. Do not let your passenger dismount the motorcycle until you say it is safe.

When You're On The Road

Wear The Proper Protection

If you're ever in a serious motorcycle crash, the best hope you have for protecting your brain is a motorcycle helmet. Always wear a helmet meeting the U.S. Department of Transportation (DOT) Federal Motor Vehicle Safety Standard (FMVSS) 218. Look for the DOT symbol on the outside back of the helmet. That is the manufacturer's way of certifying the helmet meets the DOT standard. A certified helmet also will have a permanent inside label identifying the manufacturer and providing information about the care and use of the helmet. Helmets meeting FMVSS 218 weigh around three pounds; have a thick polystyrene-foam lining; and sturdy chinstraps. ANSI or Snell labels are voluntary indicators of helmet quality. Don't leave your helmet behind on short trips because it could be a deadly mistake. Some motorcycle helmets, in addition to offering protection to your head in a crash, include plastic face shields that offer protection from wind, rain, insects, dust, and stones thrown up from cars. If your helmet doesn't have a face shield, be sure you wear goggles because eyeglasses won't keep your eyes from watering, and can easily fall off.

Arms and legs should be completely covered when riding a motorcycle, ideally by wearing leather or heavy denim. In addition to providing protection in a crash, protective gear also helps prevent dehydration. Boots or shoes should be high enough to cover your ankles, while gloves allow for a better grip and help protect your hands in the event of a crash. Wearing brightly colored clothing with reflective material will make you more visible to other vehicle drivers.

Ride Responsibly

Experienced riders know local traffic laws—and they don't take risks. Obey traffic lights, signs, speed limits, and lane markings; ride with the flow of traffic and leave plenty of room between your bike and other

> ♣ **It's A Fact!!**
> National Center for Statistics and Analysis estimates that helmets saved 1,658 motorcyclists' lives in 2006, and that 752 more could have been saved if all motorcyclists had worn helmets.
>
> Source: NHTSA, 2006.

vehicles; and always check behind you and signal before you change lanes. Remember to ride defensively. The majority of multi-vehicle motorcycle crashes generally are caused when other drivers simply didn't see the motorcyclist. Proceed cautiously at intersections and yield to pedestrians and other vehicles as appropriate. You can increase your visibility by applying reflective materials to your motorcycle and by keeping your motorcycle's headlights on at all times, even using high beams during the day.

Be Alcohol And Drug Free

Alcohol and drugs, including some prescribed medications, negatively affect your judgment, coordination, balance, throttle control, and ability to shift gears. These substances also impair your alertness and reduce your reaction time. Even when you're fully alert, it's impossible to predict what other vehicles or pedestrians are going to do. Therefore, make sure you are alcohol and drug free when you get on your motorcycle. Otherwise, you'll be heading for trouble.

Traffic Safety Facts: Motorcycles

- In 2006, 4,810 motorcyclists were killed—an increase of five percent over the 4,576 motorcyclists killed in 2005. There were 88,000 motorcyclists injured during 2006.
- Per vehicle mile traveled in 2005, motorcyclists were about 37 times more likely than passenger car occupants to die in a motor vehicle traffic crash and eight times more likely to be injured.
- Per registered vehicle, the fatality rate for motorcyclists in 2005 was 5.4 times the fatality rate for passenger car occupants. The injury rate for passenger car occupants per registered vehicle was 0.8 times the injury rate for motorcyclists.
- In 2006, 2,537 (51%) of all motorcycles involved in fatal crashes collided with another type of motor vehicle in transport. In two-vehicle crashes, 79 percent of the motorcycles involved were impacted in the front. Only 5 percent were struck in the rear.
- Motorcycles are more likely to be involved in a fatal collision with a fixed object than are other vehicles. In 2006, 25 percent of the

motorcycles involved in fatal crashes collided with fixed objects, compared to 18 percent for passenger cars, 12 percent for light trucks, and 3 percent for large trucks.

- In 2006, there were 2,226 two-vehicle fatal crashes involving a motorcycle and another type of vehicle. In 40 percent (883) of these crashes the other vehicle was turning left while the motorcycle was going straight, passing, or overtaking the vehicle. Both vehicles were going straight in 582 crashes (26%).

- In 2006, 37 percent of all motorcyclists involved in fatal crashes were speeding, compared to 23 percent for passenger car drivers, 19 percent for light-truck drivers, and 8 percent for large-truck drivers.

Licensing

One out of four motorcycle operators (25%) involved in fatal crashes in 2006 were operating their vehicles with invalid licenses at the time of the collision, while only 13 percent of drivers of passenger vehicles in fatal crashes did not have valid licenses.

Motorcycle operators involved in fatal traffic crashes were 1.2 times more likely than passenger vehicle drivers to have a previous license suspension or revocation (16% and 13%, respectively).

In 2006, 3.9 percent of the motorcycle operators involved in fatal crashes had at least one previous conviction for driving while intoxicated on their driver records, compared to 2.8 percent of passenger vehicle drivers.

Alcohol

In fatal crashes in 2006 a higher percentage of motorcycle operators had blood alcohol concentrations (BAC) of .08 grams per deciliter (g/dL) or higher than any other type of motor vehicle driver. The percentages for vehicle operators involved in fatal crashes were 27 percent for motorcycles, 23 percent for passenger cars, 24 percent for light trucks, and 1 percent for large trucks.

In 2006, 27 percent of all fatally injured motorcycle operators had BAC levels of .08 g/dL or higher. An additional 7 percent had lower alcohol levels (BAC .01 to .07 g/dL).

The percentage with BAC .08 g/dL or above was highest for fatally injured motorcycle operators among two age groups, 35–39 (41%) and 40–44 (39%) followed by ages 45–49 (34%).

Forty-one percent of the 2,007 motorcycle operators who died in single-vehicle crashes in 2006 had BAC levels of .08 g/dL or higher. Fifty-nine percent of those killed in single-vehicle crashes on weekend nights had BACs of .08 g/dL or higher.

Motorcycle operators killed in traffic crashes at night were more than three times more likely to have BAC levels of .08 g/dL or higher than those killed during the day (43% and 12%, respectively).

The reported helmet use rate for motorcycle operators with BAC levels .08 g/dL or higher killed in traffic crashes was 45 percent, compared with 66 percent for those with no alcohol (BAC = .00 g/dL).

> ♣ **It's A Fact!!**
> Forty-one percent of motorcycle operators who died in single-vehicle crashes in 2006 had blood alcohol concentration levels of .08 g/dL or higher.
>
> Source: NHTSA, 2006.

Helmet Use And Effectiveness

NHTSA estimates that helmets saved the lives of 1,658 motorcyclists in 2006. If all motorcyclists had worn helmets, an additional 752 lives could have been saved.

Helmets are estimated to be 37-percent effective in preventing fatal injuries to motorcyclists.

This means for every 100 motorcyclists killed in crashes while not wearing a helmet, 37 of them could have been saved had all 100 worn helmets.

According to NHTSA's National Occupant Protection Use Survey, a nationally representative observational survey of motorcycle helmet, seat belt, and child safety seat use, helmet use declined by 20 percentage points over five years, from 71 percent in 2000 to 51 percent in 2006. This drop is statistically significant and corresponds to a striking 70-percent increase in non-users.

Motorcycle Safety

Reported helmet use rates for fatally injured motorcyclists in 2006 were 59 percent for operators and 45 percent for passengers, compared with 58 percent and 50 percent, respectively, in 2005.

All motorcycle helmets sold in the United States are required to meet Federal Motor Vehicle Safety Standard 218, the performance standard which establishes the minimum level of protection helmets must afford each user.

In 2006, 20 states, the District of Columbia, and Puerto Rico required helmet use by all motorcycle operators and passengers. In another 26 states, only persons under a specific age, usually 18, were required to wear helmets. Four states had no laws requiring helmet use.

Chapter 31

Pedestrian Safety

Crossing Advice For Pedestrians

Each year about 5,000 pedestrians are killed and 69,000 are injured in motor vehicular crashes. Young children and the elderly are more likely to be killed or injured in a pedestrian crash than any other age group. While many are quick to blame drivers for pedestrian fatalities and injuries, the pedestrian is many times also at fault.

We are all pedestrians at one time or another, and the traffic signals, signs, and pavement markings are there to assure our safety. However, we should realize that no amount of traffic control devices will be able to protect us from ourselves if we do not pay attention to the "Signs of Safety" all around us.

Crossing Rules For Pedestrians

Always follow these steps when crossing a street:

- Always use a marked crosswalk when one is available. The bright white lines of a crosswalk remind motorists to look out for pedestrians.

About This Chapter: This chapter includes "Crossing Advice for Pedestrians," Federal Highway Administration, Pub. No. FHWA-SA-01-001, 2001; "Always Expect a Train," Federal Highway Administration, Pub. No. FHWA-SA-01-002, 2001; and excerpts from "Traffic Safety Facts: Pedestrians," National Highway Traffic Safety Administration, 2006.

- Stop at the curb, edge of road, corner, or parked vehicle before proceeding across. Look left-right-left, and if it's clear, begin crossing.
- Continue to check for traffic in all directions, especially for vehicles turning "right-on-red."
- If there is traffic, make eye contact with the driver/s so they see you, understand your intention, and stop before you start to cross.

At The Intersection Cross Only On The Proper Signal

At signalized intersections that don't have pedestrian signals, pedestrians facing a green light may cross within a crosswalk in the direction of the light, but only when it is safe to do so. At signalized intersections with pedestrian signals, its important to follow the directions given by the signals.

If there is a push button, press the button and wait for the pedestrian signal to display the "walk" indication. The "walk" signal indicates that a pedestrian facing the signal indication may proceed across the roadway in that direction. Remember to follow the basic "Crossing Rules" and check for turning vehicles.

A flashing "don't walk" signal indication means that a pedestrian shall not start to cross the roadway in the direction of the indication, but any pedestrian who has partly completed their crossing shall finish crossing or proceed to a safety island in that direction.

A steadily illuminated "don't walk" indication means a pedestrian shall not enter the roadway in the direction of the indication. Pedestrians waiting to cross must wait for the next "walk" signal.

Remember, don't take those "No Right Turn On Red" signs for granted. Always check for turning vehicles before stepping off the curb—motorists make mistakes too.

Always Expect A Train

Railroads have been an important part of transportation for over 150 years, and people from all walks of life are interested in trains.

Pedestrians should always be cautious around trains and take special care in safely crossing railroad or transit tracks. This means crossing only at designated

Pedestrian Safety

> ### 👉 Remember!! And Don't Forget
>
> - Always use sidewalks when they are available.
> - On roads without sidewalks, walk on the left side of the road, facing traffic.
> - Watch for cars backing out of parking spaces and driveways.
> - Never walk along or attempt to cross expressways, interstate highways, or turnpikes.
> - Almost 60 percent of all pedestrian fatalities occur between 6:00 p.m. and 6:00 a.m., so when walking at night, wear something retroreflective on your clothing and shoes, or just carry a flashlight. Drivers will be able to see you from 2 to 3 times further away with the retroreflective materials.
> - About 33 percent of all pedestrians killed have a blood alcohol content (BAC) of 0.1 or greater.
>
> Source: Federal Highway Administration, Pub. No. FHWA-SA-01-001.

public crossings, which are indicated by the presence of a "crossbuck" sign and a specially designed, paved crossing surface. Public crossings may also feature active warning devices such as flashing red lights. Some busy crossings even have red-and-white gates that are activated by special electronic systems that can detect the approach of a train, often before you can see it coming.

Every year, over 450 people are killed as a result of dangerous and illegal activities on or near railroad tracks and equipment. Knowing how and where to cross safely is the key to a safe walk, no matter where you're going.

Don't Ever Take a Short Cut Across Railroad Tracks

Walking along or across the railroad tracks at any place other than a public crossing is not only unsafe at any time of night or day, it's also illegal. Railroad property is private property, and it's not legal to be there if you don't work for the railroad. Railroad property typically is much wider than just the rails and the stone ballast under them—don't walk along the railroad or try to shortcut across the tracks, no matter how inviting it looks.

Modern Trains Are Quieter Than Ever Before, And Many Rail Lines Have More And Faster Trains

Always expect a train in any direction and on any track. Faster, quieter trains can arrive suddenly—almost before you can hear them coming. Don't walk along or sneak across the tracks, even if you think you're very familiar with the area and think you "know" that "trains only come through here late at night." You may be surprised.

Crossing the tracks at a public crossing is very different from crossing a street. When crossing the street, cars can be expected to stop at a STOP sign or red traffic signal, allowing you to cross. At a grade crossing, you must remember that trains will not stop for you (a freight train going 55 mph needs over a mile to stop), and any signals there are meant to alert you that a train is approaching. You should not try to cross until all trains have passed and any signals have stopped operating.

Safe walking means crossing tracks only at public crossings after checking the warning devices and looking "left, right, then left again," just as you would when crossing a street.

☞ Remember!!

Don't be tempted to "short-cut" your way home along the tracks, and don't use railroad property as a place to "hang around."

Railroad property is private property; it's a serious workplace that can be dangerous even for railroad employees who have learned the safety rules and practices required to do this very specialized work.

When you're out walking, even if it's just for recreation, remember that railroad tracks and other railroad property are no place for the public—so be safe, and stay away.

Source: Federal Highway Administration, Pub. No. FHWA-SA-01-002.

Pedestrian Safety

Traffic Safety Facts: Pedestrians

- A pedestrian is defined as any person not in or upon a motor vehicle or other vehicle.

- In 2006, 4,784 pedestrians were killed in traffic crashes in the United States—a decrease of 12 percent from the 5,449 pedestrians killed in 1996.

> ♣ **It's A Fact!!**
>
> In 2006, 4,784 pedestrians died in traffic crashes—a 12-percent decrease from the number reported in 1996.
>
> Source: NHTSA, 2006.

- On average, a pedestrian is killed in a traffic crash every 110 minutes and injured in a traffic crash every nine minutes.

- There were 61,000 pedestrians injured in traffic crashes in 2006.

- Most pedestrian fatalities in 2006 occurred in urban areas (74%), at non-intersection locations (79%), in normal weather conditions (90%), and at night (69%).

- More than two-thirds (70%) of the pedestrians killed in 2006 were males. In 2006, the male pedestrian fatality rate per 100,000 population was 2.24—more than double the rate for females (0.95 per 100,000 population). In 2006, the male pedestrian injury rate per 100,000 population was 23, compared with 17 for females.

Time Of Day And Day Of Week

Thirty-nine percent of the 369 young (under age 16) pedestrian fatalities occurred in crashes between 3 p.m. and 7 p.m.

Nearly one-half (49%) of all pedestrian fatalities occurred on Friday, Saturday, or Sunday: 16 percent, 17 percent, and 16 percent, respectively.

♣ It's A Fact!!

Pedestrian fatalities accounted for 83 percent of all nonoccupant fatalities in 2006. The 773 pedalcyclist fatalities accounted for 13 percent, and the remaining three percent were skateboard riders, roller skaters, etc.

Source: NHTSA, 2006.

Table 31.1. Nonoccupant Traffic Fatalities, 1996–2006

Year	Pedestrian	Pedalcyclists	Other	Total
1996	5,449	765	154	6,368
1997	5,321	814	153	6,288
1998	5,228	760	131	6,119
1999	4,939	754	149	5,842
2000	4,763	693	141	5,597
2001	4,901	732	123	5,756
2002	4,851	665	114	5,630
2003	4,774	629	140	5,543
2004	4,675	727	130	5,532
2005	4,892	786	186	5,854
2006	4,784	773	183	5,740

Alcohol Involvement

Alcohol involvement—either for the driver or for the pedestrian—was reported in 49 percent of the traffic crashes that resulted in pedestrian fatalities. Of the pedestrians involved, 35 percent had a blood alcohol concentration (BAC) of .08 grams per deciliter (g/dL) or higher. Of the drivers involved in fatal crashes, only 14 percent had a BAC of .08 g/dL or higher, less than one-half the rate for the pedestrians. In 6 percent of the crashes, both the driver and the pedestrian had a BAC of .08 g/dL or higher.

Part Four

Safety At Home, School, And Work

Chapter 32

How To Be Safety Savvy

Most teens think that nothing bad will ever happen to them, but the numbers tell a different story. For example, did you know that traffic accidents are the number one cause of teen deaths in the United States? Did you know that almost half of all rape victims are 18 or younger? It's important to be aware of these risks, and it's important to know that you do have the power to help keep yourself safe.

Keep reading to learn how to stay safe in relationships, at school, at home, on the road, and on the internet.

In Relationships

As a teen, you will have relationships with a lot of people. These relationships will probably include friendships and dating relationships. Most of the time, these relationships are fun and healthy, and they make us feel good about ourselves. Sometimes, though, these relationships can be unhealthy. Unhealthy relationships can cause someone to get hurt physically or emotionally. The questions and answers below will help you understand how to spot an unhealthy relationship and how to change a bad situation.

About This Chapter: Excerpted from "Safety: How to Be Safety Savvy," National Women's Health Information Center (www.girlshealth.gov), July 2007.

What is a healthy relationship?

In healthy relationships, you and your friend or the person you are dating feel good about each other and yourselves. You do activities together, like going to movies or out with other friends, and you talk to one another honestly about how you feel. These relationships can last a few weeks, a few months, or even years.

In healthy relationships, there is respect and honesty between both people. This means that you listen to each other's thoughts and opinions and accept each other's right to say no or to change your mind without giving each other a hard time. You should be able to let the other person know how you are feeling. You might disagree or argue sometimes, but in healthy relationships you should be able to talk things out to reach a solution.

What are the signs that I am in an abusive or unhealthy relationship?

There are many signs that you could be in an abusive or unhealthy relationship. Take a look at the list of warning signs below and see if any of these describe your relationship.

Your friend or the person you are going out with...

- gets angry when you talk or hang out with other friends or other dating partners.
- bosses you around.
- often gets in fights with other people or loses his or her temper.
- pressures you to have sex or to do something sexual that you don't want to do.
- uses drugs and alcohol, and tries to pressure you into doing the same thing.
- swears at you or uses mean language.
- blames you for his or her problems or tells you that it is your fault that he or she hurt you.
- insults or tries to embarrass you in front of other people.

How To Be Safety Savvy

- has physically hurt you.
- makes you feel scared of their reactions to things.
- always wants to know where you are going and who you are with.

These are just a few of the signs that you may be in an unhealthy or abusive relationship. Sometimes there are only one or two "warning signs" and sometimes there are many. If any of these signs are a part of your relationship, you should speak to a trusted adult such as a parent/guardian, teacher, doctor, nurse, or counselor right away.

How do I get out of an unhealthy or abusive relationship?

First, if you think that you are in an unhealthy relationship, you should talk to a parent/guardian, friend, counselor, doctor, teacher, coach, or other trusted person about your relationship. Tell them why you think the relationship is unhealthy and exactly what the other person has done (hit, pressured you to have sex, tried to control you). See the question "What are the signs that I am in an unhealthy or abusive relationship?" for information that can help you explain your situation to an adult. If need be, this trusted adult can help you contact your parent/guardian, counselors, school security, or even the police about the violence. With help, you can get out of an unhealthy relationship.

> **Remember!!**
> No matter why a person is violent physically, verbally/emotionally, or sexually, it is important for you to know that it is not your fault. You are not the reason for the violence. Violence is never okay.

Sometimes, leaving an abusive relationship can be dangerous, so it is very important for you to make a safety plan. Leaving the relationship will be a lot easier and safer if you have a plan.

Here are some tips on making your safety plan:

- Go to your doctor or hospital for treatment if you have been injured.
- Tell a trusted adult like a parent/guardian, counselor, doctor, teacher, or spiritual or community leader.

- Tell the person who is abusing you over the phone that you do not want to see him or her so they cannot touch you. Do this when a parent or guardian is home so you know you will be safe in your house.
- Use a diary to keep track of the date the violence happened, where you were, exactly what the person you are dating did, and exactly what effects it caused (such as bruises). This will be important if you need the police to order the person to stay away from you.
- Avoid contact with the person.
- Spend time with your other friends, and avoid walking by yourself.
- Think of safe places to go in case of an emergency, like a police station or a public place like a restaurant or mall.
- Carry a cell phone, phone card, or money for a call in case you need to call for help. Use code words on the phone that you and your family decide on ahead of time. If you are in trouble, say the code word on the phone so that your family member knows you can't talk openly and need help right away.
- Call 911 right away if you are ever afraid that the person is following you or is going to hurt you.
- Keep domestic violence hotline numbers with you in a safe place or program them into your cell phone. The 24-hour National Domestic Violence Hotline is 800-799-SAFE (800-799-7233) or 800-787-3224 (TDD).

What do I do if I am being hurt by a parent/guardian or another family member?

Sadly, there are times when different kinds of abuse happen in the home. Child abuse is when any person caring for a child fails to take care of the child, physically hurts the child, or treats the child in a sexual way. No matter what, parents, guardians, and caregivers are supposed to protect and care for their children.

If you or someone in your family is being abused at home, call the 24-hour Childhelp National Child Abuse Hotline at 800-4-A-CHILD (800-422-4453).

> ### ♣ It's A Fact!!
> ### What is rape and date rape?
>
> Rape is sex you don't agree to, including forcing a body part or object into your vagina, rectum (bottom), or mouth. Date rape is when you are raped by someone you know. Both are crimes. Rape is not about sex—it is an act of power by the rapist and it is always wrong.
>
> Date rape drugs, which often have no smell or taste, can be given to you without you knowing at parties or in a club—especially where alcohol is served. Alcohol can make you less aware of danger and make you less able to think clearly and resist sexual assault. If you are given date rape drugs, you may not be able to say "no" to unwanted sex and you may not be able to clearly remember what happened.
>
> Remember: Even if you were drinking, it is not your fault.
>
> - National Sexual Assault Hotline: 800-656-HOPE (800-656-4673). It's free, confidential, and 24 hours.

At Home

Many people feel the safest at home. Even at home, though, there are some important steps you should take to protect yourself.

- Always know who is at the door before opening it. If you're home by yourself and do not recognize the person, do not open the door.
- If you're home by yourself, do not let others know. Only your parents should know you're alone.
- If you're home by yourself and someone calls asking for your parents, tell him or her that your parents aren't available and offer to take a message.
- If a stranger wants to use your phone, tell him or her you can't help.
- If there is a stranger in your home, leave right away. Don't try to talk to the person. Go to a neighbor's house and call the police.
- Keep your doors and windows locked at all times.
- Keep emergency numbers for police, fire, and poison control handy.

- If your house has an alarm system, make sure your parents show you how to use it.

Having Fun And Staying Safe

As a teen, your family may give you more responsibilities and the chance to spend more time with your friends. This extra time with your friends may put you in new or different social situations and places. With your parents not around as much, you are making more decisions for yourself and will need to keep yourself safe. If you forget about your safety, your fun can quickly turn into danger.

New social settings like parties are a fun way for you to spend time with your friends. Most of the time parties are a safe way to hang out with your friends, but sometimes things can happen that can make a party a dangerous place to be. It's important to know what to do if a party gets out of control and how to keep yourself safe.

- Never walk away with strangers.
- Never be alone with someone who has been drinking or taking drugs.
- Don't drink alcohol or do drugs.
- Tell your parents and friends where you are going.
- Never get in a car with someone who has been drinking or doing drugs.

What can I do to develop a safety plan for different social situations?

No matter what the situation is, you can develop a plan to help keep yourself safe. Read the following list and develop your safety plan right now.

- Tell your parents where you are going, who you will be with, and when you will be back. This may sound lame, but you will be safer for doing so.
- Carry money, a phone card, or a cell phone in case you need to make an emergency phone call. Don't forget to keep emergency numbers and the phone number of a taxi service in your wallet or backpack or program them into your cell phone.
- Stay in well lit public places.

- Stick with another person or a group of your friends.
- Try to avoid strangers. If you talk to them, don't share information about yourself.
- Use code words on the phone that you and your family decide on ahead of time. If you are in trouble, say the code word so that your family member knows you can't talk openly and need to be picked up right away.

On The Road

It's late, you're tired, and all you want to do is get in the car so you can go home. But what if the driver is drunk? The answer is simple—don't get into the car. If the driver is drunk, it's going to be a long time before it is safe for him or her to drive. To protect yourself, you must find another way home. Ask someone else to drive, call your parents/guardians, call another friend, or take a cab. Some cities have safe ride programs, where you can call a number and get a free ride home. Ask your parents/guardians for help finding out if your city has a safe ride program, before you need it.

If the driver is a parent/guardian or another adult, it may be hard for you to say that you won't get in the car. Don't be afraid to ask if the person has been drinking. He or she may be surprised or offended by the question, but it's your right to have a safe ride home. If your parent/guardian is the one who is driving drunk, talk to another adult you trust.

Some of the same advice applies to taking rides from a driver who is fatigued or over-tired. Ask someone else to drive or suggest that the driver stop to rest before continuing.

You may also be driving with friends or family members who recently got their driver's licenses. New drivers may be too willing to take risks on the road, or may be careless and unsafe. Take notice and don't be afraid to speak up for your safety or to find a different way to get to where you are going.

> **Remember!!**
> You do not have to be afraid every time you leave the house. But, it is important that you take some responsibility for your own safety. Trust your instincts, pay attention to what is going on around you, and protect yourself. Remember, being safe will not take away from your fun. Being safe will make sure that you can keep having it.

What should I do if I think I'm being followed?

If you're driving and you think you're being followed, do not go home. Instead, you should keep driving until you reach a gas station, open business, or other well-lit area where you can get help, or use your cell phone to call the police.

Although it doesn't happen a lot, there have been times when a woman driving alone has been pulled over and raped by a man pretending to be a police officer. If you're signaled to pull over in a dark or deserted area, keep driving until you come to a well-lit, populated area. Let the police officer know you're planning to pull over by turning on your flashers (also called hazards) and driving at a slower speed. In some areas you may be charged for failing to heed a police officer's demands, but it's better than risking your safety.

On The Internet

The internet has opened up a whole new world for people of all ages. You can shop, plan a vacation, send a picture to a relative, talk with friends, and even do research for school. This new way of finding information and communicating does come with risks.

How can I tell if someone is telling the truth?

The scary thing is that it's really hard to tell if someone is telling the truth, especially online. There are people out there who lie about who they are and stalk young girls on the internet. For example, someone may lie and tell you that they are much younger or even older than they are. Even if you try to check on the person by reading their online profile, a person can easily lie about themselves and their age. Bottom line is that some people who use the internet can't be trusted and could hurt you.

Is IMing safe?

IMing isn't as private as you might think, so it's important to know how to stay safe and have fun too.

- Don't respond to IM's from people you don't know or IM's that look strange. It is possible to get unwanted IM's. Like e-mails, IM's can also contain viruses.

How To Be Safety Savvy

- Don't forget to sign off when you're finished and change your password regularly. This will keep others from using your IM account.
- If you get an IM that makes you feel uncomfortable, do not respond to it. Tell your parents/guardians about it.
- Never give out your screen name or password, even to your friends.

Are chat rooms safe?

Before you enter a chat, be sure you have permission from a parent or guardian to do so.

Some chat rooms are thought to be safe because the topic that is being talked about is safe and because there is a moderator leading the chat. Even if the topic is okay, some people might talk about other things that can make you uncomfortable. If you ever feel uncomfortable or in danger for any reason, leave the chat room right away and tell a parent/guardian or other trusted adult.

Is it safe to post a profile on MySpace, Friendster, or Facebook?

Many young people think the information they post on websites such as MySpace, Friendster, Facebook, blogs, or other "online communities" will only be seen by their friends. But, often, this is not the case. Anything you post online—even if it's in a "private" area—can be seen by almost anyone, including your parents/guardians, your teachers, bosses, and strangers, some of whom could be dangerous. For this reason, you should not post information about yourself. Even information that seems harmless, such as where you went to dinner last night, could be used by a stranger to find you.

You should always be careful when posting to blogs or "online communities." Scam artists have been known to use personal information from your profile to pose as a friend, in hopes that you will give them more personal information, such as your credit card or cell phone numbers. Never give out any personal information online.

- Before joining an "online community" or writing in a blog, think about who might be able to see your profile. Some sites will let only certain users see your posted content; others let everyone see postings.

- Think about keeping some control over the information you post. If you can, limit access to your page to a select group of people, such as your friends from school, your club, your team, your community groups, or your family. Keep in mind, though, this does not always mean that other people can't see your page.

- Keep your information to yourself. Don't post your full name, Social Security number, address, phone number, or bank and credit card account numbers—and don't post other people's information, either.

  Be careful about posting information that could be used to identify you or locate you at home or school. This could include the name of your school, sports team, clubs, and where you work, live, or hang out.

- Make sure your screen name doesn't say too much about you. Don't use your name, your age, or your hometown. It doesn't take a genius to combine clues to figure out who you are and where you can be found.

- Post only information that you are comfortable with others seeing—and knowing—about you. Many people can see your page, including your parents/guardians, your teachers, the police, the college you might want to apply to next year, or the job you might want to apply for in five years.

- Remember that once you post information online, you can't take it back. Even if you delete the information from a site, older versions exist on other people's computers.

- Don't post your photo. It can be changed and spread around in ways you may not be happy about.

- Don't flirt with strangers online. Because some people lie about who they really are, you never really know who you're dealing with.

- Don't meet someone you met online in person. If someone you met online wants to meet you in person, tell your parents/guardians or a trusted adult right away.

- Trust your gut if you have suspicions. If you feel threatened by someone or uncomfortable because of something online, tell your parents/guardians or an adult you trust and report it to the police and the website. You could end up protecting someone else.

How To Be Safety Savvy

- Choose your words wisely. Some websites where you can chat with your friends have rules about what you can say. You can get kicked out if you violate those rules.

What kind of online name should I choose?

You should never use your real name as your online name. By using your real name, anyone can know right away who you are and can probably find out more about you. This is especially true in chat rooms, where you can get comfortable chatting with someone and suddenly realize they know things about you.

You probably want your online name to describe who you are, but be careful about the name and words you choose. Remember when you're talking online to people you don't know well, some people may unfairly judge you by your online name. For example, if you choose a name like hotbabe13, people will get the wrong idea about you and you most likely will get unwanted e-mails from people who are just responding to your online name and not to who you really are. If you can't think of an online name to use without describing something about yourself, try using the name of a candy bar, color, or something else that's not personal. If the name is already taken, you can try adding a few numbers, for example Green123.

What do I do if someone on the internet is harassing me?

If someone on the internet sends you lots of e-mails, follows you into chat rooms, or sends you messages even after you have stopped responding,

---

♣ It's A Fact!!
What do I do if someone I talk to on the internet wants to meet in person?

Even though you may feel like you know someone you met online really well, this person is still a stranger. It's best never to meet someone you met online in person. If someone that you met online wants to meet you in person, you should tell your parents/guardians or a trusted adult right away.

then the person may be harassing you. First, tell your parents/guardians right away about the person. The next step is to try ignoring the person while you are on the internet to see if they will leave you alone and get the hint. If they continue to bother you even after you have stopped responding, then you and your parents/guardians can call your internet service provider and complain about the other person. You and your parents/guardians can also talk to the police. It is not your fault if someone starts bothering you. You and your parents/guardians can stop them from harassing you and someone else.

Chapter 33

When To Call The Police

A Guide To The Suspicious

No police department can function without the concerned assistance of responsible citizens. They are depending on you to call and tell them whenever you observe suspicious persons or actions. Some people fail to call the police simply because they are not aware of what seemingly innocent activities might be suspicious. Others may notice suspicious activity and be hesitant to call for fear of seeming a "nosy neighbor" or a "crank." Still others take it for granted that someone else has already called.

Call the police immediately about all suspicious activity... and do it yourself. Don't worry about bothering them because this is what the police are for. Don't worry about being embarrassed if your suspicions prove unfounded. Think instead about what could have happened if you had not called.

Information Most Often Needed By Police
- What happened?
- When?
- Where?
- Anyone injured?

About This Chapter: Text in this chapter is from "When To Call The Police," © 2006 National Crime Prevention Council (www.ncpc.org). Reprinted with permission.

- Vehicle tag
- Vehicle description
- Direction of travel
- Description of persons (including clothing and/or how many)

When describing suspects, notice age, race, sex, height, and weight. Compare your own weight and height with the suspects. Pick out some unique characteristics (scars, nose, jewelry, etc.) that will help you identify the suspect in the future if need be.

> ✔ **Quick Tip**
>
> For crime prevention tips, contact the National Crime Prevention Council:
>
> National Crime Prevention Council
> 2345 Crystal Drive
> Suite 500
> Arlington, VA 22202
> www.ncpc.org

What Is Suspicious?

Basically, anything that seems even slightly "out of place" or that is occurring at an unusual time of day could be criminal activity.

Some of the most obvious things to watch for and include are:

- A stranger entering your neighbor's house when it's unoccupied.
- A scream heard anywhere might mean a robbery or assault.
- Offers of merchandise at ridiculously low prices could mean stolen property.
- Any removing of accessories, license plates, or gasoline from a car should be reported.
- Persons entering or leaving a business place after hours could mean burglars.
- Anyone peering into parked cars may be looking for a car to steal, or for valuables left displayed in the car.
- The sound of breaking glass or loud explosive noises could mean an accident, burglary, or vandalism.
- Persons loitering around schools, parks, secluded areas, or in the neighborhood could be sex offenders.

When To Call The Police

- Persons loitering around the neighborhood who do not live there could be burglars looking for a target.

Some Not So Obvious Things To Watch For

Not every stranger who comes into your neighborhood is a criminal by any means. There are many perfectly legitimate door-to-door salesmen, repairmen, and servicemen moving around our neighborhood all the time. But criminals do take advantage of this by taking the guise of legitimate business representatives. After all, if a criminal looked like a criminal, no one would have any trouble spotting him. But, if you see:

- Someone going door to door in your neighborhood, watch for a while. If, after a few houses are visited, one or more of the persons tries a door to see if it is locked or goes into a back or side yard, it could be a burglar. Such action is even more suspicious, if one person remains in the front when this occurs, or if there is a car following, a few houses away. Call the police immediately; do not wait for the person to leave.

- Someone is waiting in front of a house or business if the owners are absent or… if it's a business… and the business is closed. This might be a lookout for a burglary in progress inside.

- Anyone forcing entrance to or tampering with a residence, business, or vehicle.

- A person running, especially if carrying something of value.

- Someone carrying property, if it's at an unusual hour or in an unusual place, or if the property is not wrapped as if just purchased.

- A person exhibiting unusual mental or physical symptoms may be injured, under the influence of drugs or otherwise needing medical or psychiatric assistance.

- Many people going to and from a certain residence is not suspicious, unless it occurs on a daily or very regular basis, especially during late or unusual hours. It could possibly be the scene of drugs and vice activities or a "fence" operation.

Suspicious Activities Involving Vehicles Watch For

- Any vehicle moving slowly and without lights or following a course that appears aimless or repetitive in any location, but particularly so in areas of schools, parks, and playgrounds. Occupants may be looking for places to rob or to burglarize, or they could be drug pushers or sex offenders.

- Parked, occupied vehicles that contain one or more persons, if it is an unusual hour. They could be possible lookouts for a burglary in progress, even if the occupants appear to be legitimate.

- Vehicles being loaded with valuables if parked in front of a closed business or unattended residence... even if the vehicle is a legitimate-looking commercial unit. More and more professional thieves are taking the time and trouble to customize their vehicles with special signs in order to move more freely without suspicion.

- Apparent business transactions conducted from a vehicle, especially around schools and parks. If juveniles are involved, it could mean possible drug sales.

- Persons that are being forced into vehicles... especially if they are juveniles or females... may mean a possible kidnapping.

- An abandoned vehicle parked on your block may be a stolen car.

- A "delivery man" with an alleged wrong address or asking if someone else lives there.

While some, if not all of the suspicious situations described could have innocent explanations; your police department would rather investigate a crime-prone situation than be called when it is too late. Your call could save a life, prevent an injury, or stop a criminal act. Be alert!

> ♣ **It's A Fact!!**
> **Other Unusual Activities**
>
> - Continuous "repair" operations at non-business locations could mean stolen property is being stripped, repainted, or otherwise altered.
>
> - Open or broken doors or windows at a closed business or residence whose owners are absent could mean a burglary in progress or already completed.
>
> - Unusual noises, such as gunshots, screaming, sounds of combat, abnormally barking dogs... anything suggestive of foul play or danger or illegal activity.

Chapter 34

Gun Safety

By now, you probably know what guns are and what can happen if they fall into the wrong hands. Even though guns are featured in many television shows, video games, computer games, and movies, it's important to know that real guns are dangerous. Guns are so dangerous that they can hurt or even kill someone you know—including other kids.

Being safe can keep kids, teens, and even adults from getting hurt. Many times, guns are fired by accident. All kids should know what to do if they find a gun or if they are with someone who finds a gun. Read on and learn what to do if you come into contact with a gun. Because whether you live in a big city, in the suburbs, a small town, or on a farm, it could happen.

Why Guns Aren't Fun

Even though you've seen cartoon characters get up and walk around after being shot by a gun, it's important to remember that this could only happen on television or in video games. A real gun is never a toy, and life is not a video game. Real guns use bullets that hit actual targets. If that target is an animal or a person, the bullet can rip through skin, muscles, bones,

> About This Chapter: "Gun Safety," January 2006, reprinted with permission from www.kidshealth.org. Copyright © 2006 The Nemours Foundation. This information was provided by KidsHealth, one of the largest resources online for medically reviewed health information written for parents, kids, and teens. For more articles like this one, visit www.KidsHealth.org, or www.TeensHealth.org.

and organs, doing a lot of damage. A gunshot can permanently cripple someone or even kill.

That's why you must never play with a real gun. Even if you think you're safe, anything can happen once you put your finger on the trigger. Most kids in gun accidents later say they didn't fire the gun intending to hurt anyone, yet someone got badly hurt. So never show a gun to a friend and never, ever point a gun at anyone—including yourself—even as a joke. You or your friend could end up in the hospital or worse.

It's also never funny to say you have a gun or threaten to shoot someone. These words are taken seriously and the police may be called. These pranks don't end up being fun for anyone involved.

Gun Safety At Home

Most gunshot injuries happen after kids discover loaded guns at home. In the United States, there is great debate over gun control. No one seems to agree on who should be allowed to own guns and under what conditions. But experts on all sides believe that keeping a gun in the house is a serious decision, and the gun must be kept locked up where kids can't get to it. You can tell your parents that Project ChildSafe provides free gun locks at special fairs and they can also be picked up at your local police department.

The American Academy of Pediatrics (AAP) says that the best way to prevent gun-related injuries and deaths is to remove guns from homes. However, the decision to own a gun is up to each family. Yours may have decided to keep guns in the house. Your dad may hunt, for example, or your mom may be a police officer or work in another profession where guns are required. Some families use guns for protection. But any gun can be dangerous if a kid tries to play with it.

If you come across a gun at home, you may be tempted to check it out—but don't. Eddie Eagle, a program sponsored by the National Rifle Association (NRA), teaches kids what to do when they come across a gun:

- Stop!
- Don't touch.

- Remove yourself from the area.
- Tell an adult.

Not touching the gun is very important, but don't forget to also leave the area and tell an adult. By leaving the area you can keep yourself safe in case someone else decides to touch the gun before an adult can remove it. Remember, a baby sister or brother may be strong enough to pull a trigger.

> ♣ **It's A Fact!!**
> **At A Friend's Or Neighbor's House**
> Most people don't advertise the fact that they own guns. Before you visit your friend, make sure your parents check with your friend's parents to see if they own a gun. You may already be playing at a friend's house when you learn that a gun is nearby. If your friend wants to show you the gun, say "no" and leave right away if you are close to home. Or call your parent for a ride and talk about what happened as soon as you're picked up. Don't worry about getting your friend into trouble—you will be helping to keep him or her safe.

At School

Sometimes what you hear on the news can be scary, especially if you hear about kids getting hurt at school. Once in a great while, a kid who has access to guns may use one to express anger. When that happens, no one feels safe.

One thing to remember about gun violence at school is that it doesn't happen very often. School is actually one of the safest places for you to be. Most schools never experience serious violence.

But if someone at your school threatens you or talks about bringing a gun to school, speak up. Tell an adult like a teacher, a guidance counselor, or the principal as soon as possible. If you feel awkward doing this in front of other students, ask your teacher for private time or go to the school office to talk to the principal or counselor. And tell your mom or dad. They can get in touch with the right person at your school.

Don't feel that you're being a tattletale if you tell an adult that someone is threatening you. You will not get into trouble for reporting that you don't feel safe or that another kid is doing or saying something that scares you. You may even be a hero and prevent a tragedy from happening.

Chapter 35

School And School Bus Safety

In School

School should be a place where we feel safe from harm. Many students attend schools that are very safe and comfortable places to learn. There still may be a time when you feel unsafe because other students use violence, or bullying to harm you. Sexual harassment can also make you feel unsafe. Someone is sexually harassing you if he or she says or does anything sexual to make you feel uncomfortable, including the following examples:

- Making sexual comments or jokes
- Touching you in a sexual way
- Blocking your way or cornering you in a sexual way
- Forcing you to kiss him or her or do other things that make you uncomfortable

While it is very rare for an adult at school to harass or threaten students in a sexual way, you should let a parent or guardian know right away if an adult at school makes you feel uncomfortable. You have the right to feel safe and to be respected by your classmates and adults at school. If you ever feel

> About This Chapter: This chapter begins information excerpted from "Safety: How to Be Safety Savvy," National Women's Health Institute (www.girlshealth.gov), July 2007. Additional text from the National Safety Council (www.nsc.org) is cited separately within the chapter.

> ♣ **It's A Fact!!**
>
> School bus related crashes killed 164 persons and injured an estimated 18,000 persons nationwide in 1999, according to data from the National Highway Traffic Safety Administration's Fatality Analysis Reporting System (FARS) and General Estimates System (GES).
>
> Source: © 2004 National Safety Council.

afraid or threatened, tell a teacher, school counselor, parent/guardian, or other adult you can trust.

Violence

Have you ever felt unsafe at school? Have you ever been afraid to go to school? If someone has threatened you, tell a parent/guardian or teacher immediately.

School Bus Safety Rules

"School Bus Safety Rules," © 2004 National Safety Council (www.nsc.org). Reprinted with permission.

For some 22 million students nationwide, the school day begins and ends with a trip on a school bus. Unfortunately, each year many children are injured and several are killed in school bus incidents.

Over the past six years, about 70% of the deaths in fatal school bus related crashes were occupants of vehicles other than the school bus and 20% were pedestrians. About 4% were school bus passengers and 2% were school bus drivers. Of the pedestrians killed in school bus related crashes over this period, approximately 77% were struck by the school bus. Of the people injured in school bus related crashes from 1994 through 1999, about 44% were school bus passengers, 9% were school bus drivers, and another 43% were occupants of other vehicles.

Although drivers of all vehicles are required to stop for a school bus when it is stopped to load or unload passengers, children should not rely on them

School And School Bus Safety

to do so. The National Safety Council encourages parents to teach their children these rules for getting on and off the school bus.

Rules For Getting On And Off The School Bus

Getting On The School Bus

- When waiting for the bus, stay away from traffic and avoid rough-housing or other behavior that can lead to carelessness. Do not stray onto streets, alleys, or private property.
- Line up away from the street or road as the school bus approaches.
- Wait until the bus has stopped and the door opens before stepping onto the roadway.
- Use the hand rail when stepping onto the bus.

Behavior On The Bus

- When on the bus, find a seat and sit down. Loud talking or other noise can distract the bus driver and is not allowed.
- Never put head, arms, or hands out of the window.
- Keep aisles clear—books or bags are tripping hazards and can block the way in an emergency.
- Before you reach your stop, get ready to leave by getting your books and belongings together.
- At your stop, wait for the bus to stop completely before getting up from your seat. Then, walk to the front door and exit, using the hand rail.

Getting Off The School Bus

- If you have to cross the street in front of the bus, walk at least ten feet ahead of the bus along the side of the road, until you can turn around and see the driver.
- Make sure that the driver can see you.
- Wait for a signal from the driver before beginning to cross.

- When the driver signals, walk across the road, keeping an eye out for sudden traffic changes.
- Do not cross the center line of the road until the driver has signaled that it is safe for you to begin walking.
- Stay away from the bus' rear wheels at all times.

✔ **Quick Tip**

Correct Way To Cross The Street

- Children should always stop at the curb or the edge of the road and look left, then right, and then left again before crossing.
- They should continue looking in this manner until they are safely across.
- If students' vision is blocked by a parked car or other obstacle, they should move out to where drivers can see them and they can see other vehicles—then stop, and look left-right-left again.

Source: National Safety Council. © 2004.

Chapter 36

Babysitting Basics

Maybe you've been babysitting forever and have lots of neighborhood families on your list. Maybe you just landed your very first job babysitting for your cousin. Whether you're an old pro or just starting out, babysitting is a fun way to spend some time with kids while making some extra money.

Being a babysitter is all about responsibility. As long as you're on the job, you're in charge. Not only do you have to make sure the kids are happy, you have to make sure they're safe and that their needs are taken care of.

If you're new to babysitting, check out this guide to learn how to be the best babysitter around. Been babysitting forever and think you have it down? Read on for a quick refresher course in babysitting basics, just to be sure.

Rule #1: Be Prepared

We borrowed this motto from the Boy Scouts, but we knew they wouldn't mind: It's the rule for anyone who wants to know what to do in an emergency. Most babysitting jobs are a breeze and nothing goes wrong—except maybe for an occasional fight over the last orange popsicle. But for the rare times when an emergency does happen, you want to be ready to handle it.

About This Chapter: "Babysitting Basics," June 2007, reprinted with permission from www.kidshealth.org. Copyright © 2007 The Nemours Foundation. This information was provided by KidsHealth, one of the largest resources online for medically reviewed health information written for parents, kids, and teens. For more articles like this one, visit www.KidsHealth.org, or www.TeensHealth.org.

Be sure you know the following:

Emergency Numbers: These include:

- the local emergency number (911 in most areas, but check to be sure);
- the number for the fire department that covers the area in which you're babysitting (if different from the local emergency number);
- the number for the police covering the area in which you're babysitting (if different from the local emergency number);
- the number for the local poison control center.

A lot of parents have these numbers posted by the phone or on the fridge; if not, ask.

Other Important Numbers: Ask parents to also leave these numbers:

- their cell phone or beeper number (if they have one); if not, the number for the place where they'll be;
- phone numbers for a few trusted neighbors;
- phone numbers of any relatives who live in the area;
- phone number for the children's doctor.

Ask the parent which number he or she wants you to call first. If there's a serious medical emergency, the best practice is to call 911 first, but if it's a less serious situation, such as cuts or scrapes, parents may want you to call them before calling the doctor. Find out what their preferences are. At the house, make sure the parent shows you where basic first aid supplies are in case you need them.

Medical Information: Is a child taking medicine? Do any kids have asthma? What about allergies? Parents should give you information about a child's medical conditions and how they should be handled so you know what to do in an emergency. For example, if a child is allergic to bee stings, you will want to know where the parents keep the kid's epinephrine shot (a pen-like device that gives a shot of fast-acting medication that can save the life of someone with severe allergies). The parent should also train you in how to use the shot on the child—it's easy if you know how to do it. If there

Babysitting Basics

is anything you are uncomfortable being responsible for, let the parent know before accepting the job. There are lots of babysitting jobs available—this might not be the right one for you.

Fire Safety Procedures: Every family should have a fire escape plan with more than one exit from the home, as well as a designated meeting place outside the house or apartment building. Be sure that both you and the kids know them.

Practicing fire escape plans can be a good activity for the kids and, like school fire drills, it never hurts to run through a family's escape plan regularly. Make sure the kids know not to hide; to stay low to the ground; to feel doors and doorknobs for heat before opening them; to stop, drop, and roll if their clothes or hair catch fire; and to not go back into the house for any reason. Even preschoolers can learn and understand fire safety procedures.

Make sure the smoke alarms in the home have been tested. Parents can never test them too often, and that way you know they're working for your own peace of mind. Finally, ask the child's parents to show you where they keep fire extinguishers.

Lifesaving Techniques: It's a good idea to learn basic first aid (which includes the Heimlich maneuver for choking) and infant and child CPR before embarking on your babysitting career. Discuss this with your parents, because you'll have to attend courses and make a real commitment to learn these lifesaving procedures. But it's worth the trouble to feel confident that you're trained

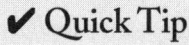

Where You Are

Sounds basic, but it's so basic that many people forget to make sure they know the correct address of the house they're in. You may know it's the green house four houses down from yours, but that won't help the fire department in an emergency. It's also easy to forget small details like a street name or number when you're caught up in an emergency—some people even forget their own address. Many parents post their address and phone number with the emergency numbers, but if you don't see it, ask. You won't sound stupid, and they'll appreciate how on the ball you are.

to help in an emergency. Plus, having these skills could give you an edge over other babysitters who don't: Parents really like these qualifications. Check with your local hospital, YMCA, or Red Cross; they often offer babysitting courses that include training in these areas. Some high schools do, too.

Rule #2: Know What To Expect

Every family you babysit for will be a little different. Having an idea of what to expect can make your babysitting experience safer and more enjoyable for everyone.

Know the family and the neighborhood. Your safety is as important as the safety of the kids you'll be watching. If this is a first babysitting job or you're just starting out, make sure you or your parents know and trust the family you're babysitting for. Give your parents the address and phone number of where you'll be, and let them know when and how you expect to be getting home.

It can feel strange to be in charge of an unfamiliar home, so help yourself feel more secure by locking windows and doors after the parents leave. Don't answer the door to strangers and never tell telephone callers that you are alone. If there is an answering machine at the house where you are babysitting, use it to screen callers you don't know.

Know the kids you'll be babysitting. Of course, babysitting a 2-month-old baby is pretty different from babysitting a 10-year-old kid. Know the ages of the kids ahead of time. If you don't feel comfortable babysitting a newborn, for example, then don't take the job. You need to feel you're in control, and if you're unsure, it's better to wait for the next job.

Know how many kids you'll be babysitting. You think you're babysitting for the Simon twins, but when you arrive you also see their two 5-year-old cousins and a 7-year-old friend. Perhaps you're not ready to take care of five small kids at once. Most adults aren't! So ask ahead of time how many kids there will be—including friends and relatives. If you arrive and there are too many kids, say something to the parents. They may let you call a friend to help, or they may call and ask another babysitter to come and join you. And if you get loaded up with too many kids again, cross the family off your babysitting list.

Babysitting Basics

Know How You'll Get Home: Make sure that you have a ride home from your babysitting job. Don't wait until the last minute—check before you leave your house to make sure that a parent or sibling can pick you up at the right time. If the parents you're babysitting agree to take you home, that's great, but don't assume that they can or will. If you live within walking distance but it's after dark when the parents get back, ask someone to walk you home.

Rule #3: Stay Focused On The Kids At All Times

It doesn't matter how short or how long your babysitting assignment is. As long as you're in charge of kids, your job is to babysit—and nothing else. Naturally, this doesn't mean that you can't go to the bathroom. But otherwise, you should be with the kids every minute they are awake. It can be pretty tempting to leave them in one room while you watch TV in another room, but kids can get into trouble pretty quickly. Keeping an eye on everyone means you'll be less likely to need those emergency numbers.

This rule is especially important if you're giving kids a bath. Never leave a child unattended in the tub, even for a minute; small children can drown in as little as an inch of water. If the phone rings, let the answering machine pick it up or let the caller call back. And if you have a bashful kid who's embarrassed to be naked, draw the shower curtain to give him or her some privacy. You could also bring a book or magazine into the bathroom with you and "read" while the child takes a bath, covering your face if you have to.

♣ **It's A Fact!!**
Eating, Bathing,
Homework, And Other Fun Stuff

You need to know exactly what's expected of you. It's not unusual for parents to want you to feed the kids, give them a bath, or help them with their homework before you put them to bed. Plus, make sure you know if the kids have any special requirements. For example, parents should tell you about any food allergies or nutrition needs a child has before you start whipping up dinner.

Once the kids are in bed, you are free to do what you want—within the parents' guidelines. Most parents will say it's fine to watch TV or movies or to talk on the phone. Just remember to keep calls from the family's phone local and short, in case the parents try to call and check on the kids.

Some parents may say it's fine to have a friend come over after the kids are asleep, but you should definitely ask if it's OK to have a friend visit beforehand to avoid problems. If you don't ask and the parents come home early and find you and your pal hanging out, they may not ask you to babysit again. Some parents may think you're too distracted by the friend to focus on the kids; others may not like the thought of someone they don't know in the house. Just as you want to know what to expect, so do they.

Even if a child is in bed, be aware that he or she may need you. It's a good idea to check on the kids every half hour or so. Don't get so involved in other activities that you miss a child's call or an unusual noise. Nightmares, a drink of water—anything that wakes a kid and gets him or her out of bed is something you need to be there for.

After a night of successful babysitting, you'll have more than a heavier wallet and a great referral. You'll have the satisfaction of a job well done—and you'll have learned more about what's involved in taking care of kids.

Chapter 37

Fire Safety And Escape Planning

Escape Planning

More than 4,000 Americans die each year in fires, and approximately 20,000 are injured. Deaths resulting from failed emergency escapes are particularly avoidable. The United States Fire Administration (USFA) believes that having a sound escape plan will greatly reduce fire deaths and protect you and your family's safety if a fire occurs.

Have A Sound Fire Escape Plan

In the event of a fire, remember—time is the biggest enemy and every second counts. Escape plans help you get out of your home quickly. In less than 30 seconds a small flame can get completely out of control and turn into a major fire. It only takes minutes for a house to fill with thick black smoke and become engulfed in flames.

Practice Escaping From Every Room In The Home: Practice escape plans every month. The best plans have two ways to get out of each room. If the

---

About This Chapter: This chapter includes excerpts from the following publications produced by the U.S. Fire Administration: "Escape Planning: Get Out Safely," December 2007; "Smoke Alarms," January 2008; "Bedroom Fire Safety," November 2007; "Summer Fire Safety," December 2007; "Winter Fires: Safety Tips for the Home," December 2007; "High-Rise Residents," December 2006; "Fire Safety Beyond the City Limits," December 2006; "Live Safely in Your Manufactured Home," December 2006; "Electrical Fire Safety," December 2006; "Cooking Fire Safety," November 2007; and "Holiday Fire Safety," December 2007.

primary way is blocked by fire or smoke, you will need a second way out. A secondary route might be a window onto an adjacent roof or using an Underwriter's Laboratory (UL) listed collapsible ladder for escape from upper story windows. Make sure that windows are not stuck, screens can be taken out quickly, and that security bars can be properly opened. Also, practice feeling your way out of the house in the dark or with your eyes closed.

Security Bars Require Special Precautions: Security bars may help to keep your family safe from intruders, but they can also trap you in a deadly fire. Windows and doors with security bars must have quick release devices to allow them to be opened immediately in an emergency. Make sure everyone in the family understands and practices how to properly operate and open locked or barred doors and windows.

Immediately Leave The Home: When a fire occurs, do not waste any time saving property. Take the safest exit route, but if you must escape through smoke, remember to crawl low, under the smoke and keep your mouth covered. The smoke contains toxic gases which can disorient you or, at worst, overcome you.

Never Open Doors That Are Hot To The Touch: When you come to a closed door, use the back of your hand to feel the top of the door, the doorknob, and the crack between the door and door frame to make sure that fire is not on the other side. If it feels hot, use your secondary escape route. Even if the door feels cool, open it carefully. Brace your shoulder against the door and open it slowly. If heat and smoke come in, slam the door and make sure it is securely closed, then use your alternate escape route.

Designate A Meeting Place Outside And Take Attendance: Designate a meeting location away from the home, but not necessarily across the street. For example, meet under a specific tree or at the end of the driveway or front sidewalk to make sure everyone has gotten out safely and no one will be hurt looking for someone who is already safe. Designate one person to go to a neighbor's home to phone the fire department.

Once Out, Stay Out: Remember to escape first, then notify the fire department using the 911 system or proper local emergency number in your area. Never go back into a burning building for any reason. Teach children

Fire Safety And Escape Planning

not to hide from firefighters. If someone is missing, tell the firefighters. They are equipped to perform rescues safely.

Smoke Alarms

In the event of a fire, a smoke alarm can save your life and those of your loved ones. They are a very important means of preventing house and apartment fire fatalities by providing an early warning signal—so you and your family can escape. Smoke alarms are one of the best safety devices you can buy and install to protect yourself, your family, and your home.

Install smoke alarms on every level of your home, including the basement. Many fatal fires begin late at night or in the early morning. For extra safety, install smoke alarms both inside and outside sleeping areas. Since smoke and many deadly gases rise, installing your smoke alarms at the proper level will provide you with the earliest warning possible. Always follow the manufacturer's installation instructions.

> ✔ **Quick Tip**
>
> Pick a holiday or your birthday and replace the batteries each year on that day. If your smoke alarm starts making a "chirping" noise, replace the batteries and reset it.
>
> Source: "Smoke Alarms," January 2008.

Bedroom Fire Safety

Bedrooms are a common area of fire origin. Nearly 600 lives are lost to fires that start in bedrooms. Many of these fires are caused by misuse or poor maintenance of electrical devices, such as overloading extension cords or using portable space heaters too close to combustibles. Many other bedroom fires are caused by children who play with matches and lighters, careless smoking among adults, and arson.

Kids And Fire: A Bad Match

Children are one of the highest risk groups for deaths in residential fires. At home, children usually play with fire—lighters, matches and other ignitables—in bedrooms, in closets, and under beds. These are "secret" places where there are a lot of things that catch fire easily. Children of all ages set over 35,000 fires annually.

Appliances Need Special Attention

Bedrooms are the most common room in the home where electrical fires start. Electrical fires are a special concern during winter months which call for more indoor activities and increases in lighting, heating, and appliance use.

- Do not trap electric cords against walls where heat can build up.
- Take extra care when using portable heaters. Keep bedding, clothes, curtains and other combustible items at least three feet away from space heaters.
- Only use lab-approved electric blankets and warmers. Check to make sure the cords are not frayed.

Summer Fire Safety

Every year Americans look forward to summer vacations, camping, family reunions, picnics, and the Fourth of July. Summertime, however, also brings fires and injuries due to fireworks and outdoor grills. Annually more than 8,000 Americans are injured by fireworks and grill fires. More than half these injuries occur during the first week of July.

U.S. Fire Administration's National Fire Data Center estimates that yearly outside cooking grills cause more than 6,000 fires, over five fatalities, more than 170 injuries, and $35 million in property loss. Gas grills alone cause over 2,700 fires, 80 injuries, and $11 million dollars damage. Most of the gas grill fires and explosions were caused by gas leaks, blocked tubes, and overfilled propane tanks.

Fireworks Safety

- The best way to enjoy fireworks is to visit public fireworks displays put on by professionals who know how to safely handle fireworks.
- If you plan to use fireworks, make sure they are legal in your area.
- Never light fireworks indoors or near dry grass.

Fire Safety And Escape Planning

- Always have a bucket of water or a fire extinguisher nearby. Know how to operate the fire extinguisher properly.
- Do not wear loose clothing while using fireworks.
- Stand several feet away from lit fireworks. If a devise does not go off, do not stand over it to investigate it. Put it out with water and dispose of it.
- Always read the directions and warning labels on fireworks. If a devise is not marked with the contents, direction, and a warning label, do not light it.
- Supervise children around fireworks at all times.

Campfire Safety

- Build campfires where they will not spread, away from dry grass and leaves.
- Keep campfires small, and don't let them get out of hand.
- Keep plenty of water and a shovel around to douse the fire when you're done. Stir it and douse it again with water.
- Never leave campfires unattended.

Winter Fires: Safety Tips For The Home

The high cost of home heating fuels and utilities have caused many Americans to search for alternate sources of home heating. The use of woodburning stoves is growing, and space heaters are selling rapidly or coming out of storage. Fireplaces are burning wood and manmade logs.

All these methods of heating may be acceptable. They are, however, a major contributing factor in residential fires. Many of these fires can be prevented by following appropriate precautions. Visit the U.S. Fire Administration online (www.usfa.dhs.gov) for safety tips.

High-Rise Residents

A key to fire safety for those who live and work in these special structures is to practice specific high-rise fire safety and prevention behaviors. The United States Fire Administration (USFA) would like you to know there are simple fire safety steps you can take to prevent the loss of life and property in high-rise fires.

> ✔ **Quick Tip**
> **Keep Fireplaces And Wood Stoves Clean**
>
> - Have your chimney or wood stove inspected and cleaned annually by a certified chimney specialist.
> - Clear the area around the hearth of debris, decorations, and flammable materials.
> - Always use a metal mesh screen with fireplaces. Leave glass doors open while burning a fire.
> - Install stovepipe thermometers to help monitor flue temperatures.
> - Keep air inlets on wood stoves open, and never restrict air supply to fireplaces. Otherwise you may cause creosote buildup that could lead to a chimney fire.
> - Use fire-resistant materials on walls around wood stoves.
>
> Source: "Fireplace and Home Fire Safety," U.S. Fire Administration, November 2007.

Be Prepared For A High-Rise Fire Emergency

- Never lock fire exits or doorways, halls, or stairways. Fire doors provide a way out during the fire and slow the spread of fire and smoke. Never prop stairway or other fire doors open.
- Learn your building evacuation plan. Make sure everyone knows what to do if the fire alarm sounds. Plan and practice your escape plan together.
- Be sure your building manager posts evacuation plans in high traffic areas, such as lobbies.
- Learn the sound of your building's fire alarm and post emergency numbers near all telephones.
- Know who is responsible for maintaining the fire safety systems. Make sure nothing blocks these devices and promptly report any sign of damage or malfunction to the building management.

If The Door Is Warm To The Touch: Before you try to leave your apartment or office, feel the door with the back of your hand. If the door feels warm to the touch, do not attempt to open it. Stay in your apartment.

If The Door Is Not Warm To The Touch: If you do attempt to open the door, brace your body against the door while staying low to the floor and slowly open it a crack. What you are doing is checking for the presence of smoke or fire in the hallway. If there is no smoke in the hallway or stairwells, follow your building's evacuation plan. If you encounter smoke or flames on your way out, immediately return to your apartment.

Fire Safety Beyond The City Limits

If you live in the rural-urban interface, the point where homes meet combustible vegetation, you must increase your role to protect lives and property in your community beyond the city limits. Once a fire starts outdoors in a rural area, it is often hard to control. Wildland firefighters are trained to protect natural resources, not homes and buildings.

Many homes are located far from fire stations. The result is longer emergency response times. Within a matter of minutes, an entire home may be destroyed by fire. Limited water supply in rural areas can make fire suppression difficult. Homes may be secluded and surrounded by woods, dense brush, and combustible vegetation that fuel fires.

Live Safely In Your Manufactured Home

During a typical year, manufactured homes account for 17,700 fires, hundreds of deaths and $155 million in property losses. Manufactured homes have a fire death rate per 100,000 housing units, 32–50 percent higher than the rate for other dwellings.

Electrical system malfunctions and heating fires are the leading causes of fire in manufactured homes. Together, they account for one-third of manufactured housing fires. Electrical distribution fires occur nearly twice as often in manufactured homes as in one- and two-family dwellings.

Safety Precautions

- Have a minimum of two smoke alarms installed in your home regardless of sleeping space arrangements.

- Maintain your home heating system by having it serviced at least once a year by a professional.

- Do not store combustibles or flammables near heat sources.

- Never overload outlets, extension cords, or electrical circuits. If the circuit breaker trips or fuses blow, immediately call a licensed electrician to check your system.

> ✔ **Quick Tip**
> If smokers have visited, be sure to check the floor and around chair cushions for ashes that may have been dropped accidentally.
>
> Source: "Careless Smoking," U.S. Fire Administration, January 2007.

- Have an escape plan and practice escape routes with your family.

- Space heaters need their space. Do not place portable space heaters close to drapes, clothing, or other combustible materials.

- Install skirting material to keep leaves and other debris and combustible items from blowing under your manufactured home.

- When considering a new home, ask if residential sprinklers are available as an option.

- If there is a fire—get out immediately, go to a neighbor's and notify the fire department using the 911 system or the proper local emergency number in your area.

Electrical Fire Safety

During a typical year, home electrical problems account for 67,800 fires, 485 deaths, and $868 million in property losses. Home electrical wiring causes twice as many fires as electrical appliances. December is the most dangerous month for electrical fires. Fire deaths are highest in winter months which call for more indoor activities and increase in lighting, heating, and appliance use. Most electrical wiring fires start in the bedroom.

Safety Precautions

- Frayed wires can cause fires. Replace all worn, old, or damaged appliance cords immediately.

Fire Safety And Escape Planning

- Use electrical extension cords wisely and don't overload them.
- Keep electrical appliances away from wet floors and counters; pay special care to electrical appliances in the bathroom and kitchen.
- When buying electrical appliances look for products which meet the Underwriter's Laboratory (UL) standard for safety.
- Don't allow children to play with or around electrical appliances like space heaters, irons and hair dryers.
- Keep clothes, curtains, and other potentially combustible items at least three feet from all heaters.
- If an appliance has a three-prong plug, use it only in a three-slot outlet. Never force it to fit into a two-slot outlet or extension cord.
- Never overload extension cords or wall sockets. Immediately shut off, then professionally replace, light switches that are hot to the touch and lights that flicker. Use safety closures to "child-proof" electrical outlets.
- Check your electrical tools regularly for signs of wear. If the cords are frayed or cracked, replace them. Replace any tool if it causes even small electrical shocks, overheats, shorts out, or gives off smoke or sparks.

Cooking Fire Safety

It's a recipe for serious injury or even death to wear loose clothing (especially hanging sleeves), walk away from a cooking pot on the stove, or leave flammable materials, such as potholders or paper towels, around the stove. Whether you are cooking the family holiday dinner or a snack, practicing safe cooking behaviors will help keep you safe.

Safe Cooking Behaviors

- Always use cooking equipment tested and approved by a recognized testing facility.
- Follow manufacturers' instructions and code requirements when installing and operating cooking equipment.

- Plug microwave ovens and other cooking appliances directly into an outlet. Never use an extension cord for a cooking appliance, as it can overload the circuit and cause a fire.

- The leading cause of fires in the kitchen is unattended cooking.

- Stay in the kitchen when you are frying, grilling, or broiling food. If you leave the kitchen for even a short period of time, turn off the stove.

- If you are simmering, baking, roasting, or boiling food, check it regularly, remain in the home while food is cooking, and use a timer to remind you that you're cooking.

- Stay alert. To prevent cooking fires, you have to be alert. You won't be if you are sleepy, have been drinking alcohol, or have taken medicine that makes you drowsy.

- Keep anything that can catch fire—potholders, oven mitts, wooden utensils, paper or plastic bags, food packaging, towels, or curtains—away from your stove top.

- Keep the stove top, burners, and oven clean.

- Keep pets off cooking surfaces and nearby counter tops to prevent them from knocking things onto the burner.

- Wear short, close-fitting, or tightly rolled sleeves when cooking. Loose clothing can dangle onto stove burners and catch fire if it comes into contact with a gas flame or electric burner. If your clothes catch fire, stop, drop, and roll. Stop immediately, drop to the ground, and cover face with hands. Roll over and over or back and forth to put out the fire. Immediately cool the burn with cool water for three to five minutes and then seek emergency medical care.

Use Equipment For Intended Purposes Only: Cook only with equipment designed and intended for cooking, and heat your home only with equipment designed and intended for heating. There is additional danger of fire, injury, or death if equipment is used for a purpose for which it was not intended.

Fire Safety And Escape Planning

> ✔ **Quick Tip**
>
> **Prevent Scalds And Burns**
> - To prevent spills due to overturn of appliances containing hot food or liquids, use the back burner when possible and/or turn pot handles away from the stove's edge. All appliance cords need to be kept coiled and away from counter edges.
> - Use oven mitts or potholders when moving hot food from ovens, microwave ovens, or stove tops. Never use wet oven mitts or potholders as they can cause scald burns.
> - Replace old or worn oven mitts.
> - Treat a burn right away, putting it in cool water. Cool the burn for three to five minutes. If the burn is bigger than your fist or if you have any questions about how to treat it, seek medical attention right away.
>
> **Install And Use Microwave Ovens Safely**
> - Place or install the microwave oven at a safe height, within easy reach of all users. The face of the person using the microwave oven should always be higher than the front of the microwave oven door. This is to prevent hot food or liquid from spilling onto a user's face or body from above and to prevent the microwave oven itself from falling onto a user.
> - Never use aluminum foil or metal objects in a microwave oven. They can cause a fire and damage the oven.
> - Open heated food containers slowly away from the face to avoid steam burns. Hot steam escaping from the container or food can cause burns.
>
> Source: "Cooking Fire Safety," U.S. Fire Administration, November 2007.

Holiday Fire Safety

Each year fires occurring during the holiday season claim the lives of over 400 people, injure 1,650 more, and cause over $990 million in damage. According to the United States Fire Administration (USFA), there are simple life-saving steps you can take to ensure a safe and happy holiday. By following some of the outlined precautionary tips, individuals can greatly reduce their chances of becoming a holiday fire casualty.

Preventing Christmas Tree Fires: Special fire safety precautions need to be taken when keeping a live tree in the house. A burning tree can rapidly fill a room with fire and deadly gases. Needles on fresh trees should be green and hard to pull back from the branches, and the needle should not break if the tree has been freshly cut. Old trees can be identified by bouncing the tree trunk on the ground. If many needles fall off, the tree has been cut too long, has probably dried out, and is a fire hazard.

Do not place your tree close to a heat source, including a fireplace or heat vent. The heat will dry out the tree, causing it to be more easily ignited by heat, flame or sparks. When the tree becomes dry, discard it promptly. The best way to dispose of your tree is by taking it to a recycling center or having it hauled away by a community pick-up service.

Holiday Lights: Inspect holiday lights each year for frayed wires, bare spots, gaps in the insulation, broken or cracked sockets, and excessive kinking or wear before putting them up. Do not overload electrical outlets. Do not link more than three light strands, unless the directions indicate it is safe. Do not leave holiday lights on unattended.

Holiday Decorations: Use only nonflammable decorations. never put wrapping paper in a fireplace. It can throw off dangerous sparks and produce a chemical buildup in the home that could cause an explosion. If you are using a metallic or artificial tree, make sure it is flame retardant.

Candle Care: Avoid using lit candles: If you do use them, make sure they are in stable holders and place them where they cannot be easily knocked down. Never put lit candles on a tree.

Chapter 38

About Fire Extinguishers

There are basically four different types or classes of fire extinguishers, each of which extinguishes specific types of fire. Newer fire extinguishers use a picture/labeling system to designate which types of fires they are to be used on. Older fire extinguishers are labeled with colored geometrical shapes with letter designations.

Additionally, Class A and Class B fire extinguishers have a numerical rating which is based on tests conducted by Underwriter's Laboratories that are designed to determine the extinguishing potential for each size and type of extinguisher.

Fire Extinguisher Ratings

Class A extinguishers will put out fires in ordinary combustibles, such as wood and paper. The numerical rating for this class of fire extinguisher refers to the amount of water the fire extinguisher holds and the amount of fire it will extinguish.

Class B extinguishers should be used on fires involving flammable liquids, such as grease, gasoline, oil, etc. The numerical rating for this class of fire extinguisher states the approximate number of square feet of a flammable liquid fire that a non-expert person can expect to extinguish.

About This Chapter: "All You Ever Wanted to Know about Fire Extinguishers," © 2008 Hanford Fire Department. Reprinted with permission.

Class C extinguishers are suitable for use on electrically energized fires. This class of fire extinguishers does not have a numerical rating. The presence of the letter "C" indicates that the extinguishing agent is non-conductive.

Class D extinguishers are designed for use on flammable metals and are often specific for the type of metal in question. There is no picture designator for Class D extinguishers. These extinguishers generally have no rating nor are they given a multi-purpose rating for use on other types of fires.

Types Of Fire Extinguishers

Dry chemical extinguishers are usually rated for multiple purpose use. They contain an extinguishing agent and use a compressed, non-flammable gas as a propellant.

Halon extinguishers contain a gas that interrupts the chemical reaction that takes place when fuels burn. These types of extinguishers are often used to protect valuable electrical equipment since they leave no residue to clean up. Halon extinguishers have a limited range, usually four to six feet. The initial application of Halon should be made at the base of the fire, even after the flames have been extinguished.

♣ **It's A Fact!!**
Multi-Class Ratings
Many extinguishers available today can be used on different types of fires and will be labeled with more than one designator, for example A-B, B-C, or A-B-C. Make sure that if you have a multi-purpose extinguisher it is properly labeled.

Water extinguishers contain water and compressed gas and should only be used on Class A (ordinary combustibles) fires.

Carbon dioxide (CO_2) extinguishers are most effective on Class B and C (liquids and electrical) fires. Since the gas disperses quickly, these extinguishers are only effective from three to eight feet. The carbon dioxide is stored as a compressed liquid in the extinguisher; as it expands, it cools the surrounding air. The cooling will often cause ice to form around the "horn" where the gas is expelled from the extinguisher. Since the fire could re-ignite, continue to apply the agent even after the fire appears to be out.

About Fire Extinguishers

How To Use A Fire Extinguisher

Even though extinguishers come in a number of shapes and sizes, they all operate in a similar manner. Here's an easy acronym for fire extinguisher use: PASS—Pull, Aim, Squeeze, and Sweep.

Pull the pin at the top of the extinguisher that keeps the handle from being accidentally pressed.

Aim the nozzle toward the base of the fire.

Stand approximately eight feet away from the fire and squeeze the handle to discharge the extinguisher. If you release the handle, the discharge will stop.

Sweep the nozzle back and forth at the base of the fire. After the fire appears to be out, watch it carefully since it may re-ignite.

Chapter 39

The Dangers Of Carbon Monoxide

Each year in America, unintentional carbon monoxide poisoning claims more than 500 lives and sends another 15,000 people to hospital emergency rooms for treatment.

The United States Fire Administration (USFA) and the National Association of Home Builders (NAHB) would like you to know that there are simple steps you can take to protect yourself from deadly carbon monoxide fumes.

What is carbon monoxide?

Carbon monoxide is an odorless, colorless, and toxic gas. Because it is impossible to see, taste, or smell the toxic fumes, CO can kill you before you are aware it is in your home. At lower levels of exposure, CO causes mild effects that are often mistaken for the flu. These symptoms include headaches, dizziness, disorientation, nausea, and fatigue. The effects of CO exposure can vary greatly from person to person depending on age, overall health, and the concentration and length of exposure.

Where does carbon monoxide come from?

CO gas can come from several sources: gas-fired appliances, charcoal grills, wood-burning furnaces, or fireplaces and motor vehicles.

About This Chapter: From "Exposing an Invisible Killer: The Dangers of Carbon Monoxide," U.S. Fire Administration, December 2006.

Who is at risk?

Everyone is at risk for CO poisoning. Medical experts believe that unborn babies, infants, children, senior citizens, and people with heart or lung problems are at even greater risk for CO poisoning.

What actions do I take if my carbon monoxide alarm goes off?

What you need to do if your carbon monoxide alarm goes off depends on whether anyone is feeling ill or not.

If no one is feeling ill take these steps:

- Silence the alarm.

- Turn off all appliances and sources of combustion (that is furnace and fireplace).

- Ventilate the house with fresh air by opening doors and windows.

- Call a qualified professional to investigate the source of the possible CO buildup.

If illness is a factor take these steps:

- Evacuate all occupants immediately.

- Determine how many occupants are ill and determine their symptoms.

- Call your local emergency number and when relaying information to the dispatcher, include the number of people feeling ill.

- Do not re-enter the home without the approval of a fire department representative.

- Call a qualified professional to repair the source of the CO.

♣ **It's A Fact!!**

Every year, more than 500 people die in the U.S. from accidental CO poisoning.

CO is found in combustion fumes, such as those produced by small gasoline engines, stoves, generators, lanterns, and gas ranges, or by burning charcoal and wood. CO from these sources can build up in enclosed or partially enclosed spaces. People and animals in these spaces can be poisoned and can die from breathing CO.

Excerpted from "Preventing Carbon Monoxide Poisoning After an Emergency," Centers for Disease Control and Prevention, July 2006.

The Dangers Of Carbon Monoxide

How can I protect myself from CO poisoning?

- Install at least one UL (Underwriters Laboratories) listed carbon monoxide alarm with an audible warning signal near the sleeping areas and outside individual bedrooms. Carbon monoxide alarms measure levels of CO over time and are designed to sound an alarm before an average, healthy adult would experience symptoms. It is very possible that you may not be experiencing symptoms when you hear the alarm. This does not mean that CO is not present.

- Have a qualified professional check all fuel burning appliances, furnaces, venting and chimney systems at least once a year.

- Never use your range or oven to help heat your home and never use a charcoal grill or hibachi in your home or garage.

- Never keep a car running in a garage. Even if the garage doors are open, normal circulation will not provide enough fresh air to reliably prevent a dangerous buildup of CO.

- When purchasing an existing home, have a qualified technician evaluate the integrity of the heating and cooking systems, as well as the sealed spaces between the garage and house. The presence of a carbon monoxide alarm in your home can save your life in the event of CO buildup.

♣ **It's A Fact!!**
How To Recognize CO Poisoning

Exposure to CO can cause loss of consciousness and death. The most common symptoms of CO poisoning are headache, dizziness, weakness, nausea, vomiting, chest pain, and confusion. People who are sleeping or who have been drinking alcohol can die from CO poisoning before ever having symptoms.

Excerpted from "Preventing Carbon Monoxide Poisoning After an Emergency," Centers for Disease Control and Prevention, July 2006.

Chapter 40

Poison Prevention Tips

Home Safety Council research shows that poisoning is the second leading cause of unintentional injury related death in the home. According to the American Association of Poison Control Centers (AAPCC) more than 92 percent of the 2.4 million poison exposures reported in the latest year studied occurred in the home. Yet, the Home Safety Council found that most families are not taking the appropriate precautions to reduce the risk of poison exposure.

Poison prevention is for everyone, not just children. The Home Safety Council's poisoning prevention advice can help individuals and families keep their homes safer from poisonous and toxic products, chemicals, and gases, regardless of the ages of the occupants. Homes with young children need to take extra precautions. Follow these guidelines to keep your family safe from poison exposures at home:

Be Prepared

- Know to call 800-222-1222 if someone takes poison. This number will connect you to emergency help in your area.

- Keep the number by every phone.

About This Chapter: "Think Safe Be Safe: Poison Prevention Tips," © 2008 Home Safety Council (www.homesafetycouncil.org). Reprinted with permission.

- Carbon monoxide (CO) is a deadly gas that you cannot see or smell. The gas collects when fuels are burned.
- Have a service person check heaters, stoves, and fireplaces every year to see that they work well.
- Have a carbon monoxide (CO) detector near the bedrooms. This will tell you if the gas level is too high.
- Push the "test" button on the detector so everyone will know the sound it makes.
- Know the things in your home that are poisons.
- Look at the labels for the words "Caution," "Warning," or "Danger" on the box or bottle. Read the labels and follow directions when using these.

Protect Young Children

- Take all medicines and medical supplies out of purses, pockets, and drawers.
- Put them in a cabinet with a child safety lock.
- Have child safety caps on all chemicals, medications, and cleaning products.
- Lock all dangerous items and products in a cabinet. Cosmetics (make-up) can be poison too.
- Keep all dangerous products in the bottle or package they came in, with the labels on.
- Store all dangerous products away from food and drinks.
- Keep each family member's medicines in a separate place, so they don't get mixed up.

In The Bathroom

- Keep all chemicals, cosmetics (make-up), medicines and medical supplies, and cleaning products in the containers they came in with the labels on.

Poison Prevention Tips

- Have a medicine cabinet you can lock.
- Flush old or unwanted medicines down the toilet.[1]

In The Garage And Storage Areas

- Chemicals, fuels (such as gasoline), car fluids (such as antifreeze), pesticides (such as bug killers), and lawn and garden products (such as fertilizer) are poison.
- Close the lid and put all dangerous products away after using them.
- Store them where children cannot reach them.
- Close and put away dangerous products after using them.
- Clean up spills as soon as they happen.

> ✔ **Quick Tip**
>
> To safely dispose of all unused or expired prescription drugs, take the drugs out of their original containers, mix them with undesirable items (coffee grounds or kitty litter) and put them in watertight and unmarked containers, like empty cans or bags that can be sealed shut. Throw the containers in the trash.

When Using Motors

- Carbon monoxide (CO) is a deadly gas that you cannot see or smell. The gas collect when fuels are burned.
- Never run the car inside the garage, even with the door open.
- Use portable generators outside only. Do not use it inside your home or garage.
- Use a barbecue grill outside only. Do not use it in your home or garage.

Editor's Note

1. The U.S. Food and Drug Administration offers additional details about the safe disposal of unused medications at http://www.fda.gov/updates/drug_disposal062308.html.

Chapter 41

Electrical And Power Outage Safety

Electrical Safety

Whenever you work with power tools or on electrical circuits there is a risk of electrical hazards, especially electrical shock. Anyone can be exposed to these hazards at home or at work.

Coming in contact with an electrical voltage can cause current to flow through the body, resulting in electrical shock and burns. Serious injury or even death may occur. As a source of energy, electricity is used without much thought about the hazards it can cause. Because electricity is a familiar part of our lives, it often is not treated with enough caution.

How is an electrical shock received?

An electrical shock is received when electrical current passes through the body. Current will pass through the body in a variety of situations. Whenever two wires are at different voltages, current will pass between them if they are connected. Your body can connect the wires if you touch both of them at the same time. Current will pass through your body.

About This Chapter: This chapter includes excerpts from "Electrical Safety: Safety and Health for Electrical Trades, Student Manual," National Institute for Occupational Safety and Health, 2002; and excerpts from "What You Need to Know When the Power Goes Out Unexpectedly," Centers for Disease Control and Prevention, January 2008.

In most household wiring, the black wires and the red wires are at 120 volts. The white wires are at zero volts because they are connected to ground. The connection to ground is often through a conducting ground rod driven into the earth. The connection can also be made through a buried metal water pipe. If you come in contact with an energized black wire—and you are also in contact with the neutral white wire—current will pass through your body. You will receive an electrical shock.

> ♣ **It's A Fact!!**
> Electrocution is the third leading cause of work-related deaths among 16- and 17-year-olds, after motor vehicle deaths and workplace homicide. Electrocution is the cause of 12% of all workplace deaths among young workers.
>
> Source: National Institute for Occupational Safety and Health, 2002.

If you are in contact with a live wire or any live component of an energized electrical device—and also in contact with any grounded object—you will receive a shock.

Your risk of receiving a shock is greater if you stand in a puddle of water. But you don't even have to be standing in water to be at risk. Wet clothing, high humidity, and perspiration also increase your chances of being electrocuted. Of course, there is always a chance of electrocution, even in dry conditions.

You can even receive a shock when you are not in contact with an electrical ground. Contact with both live wires of a 240-volt cable will deliver a shock. (This type of shock can occur because one live wire may be at +120 volts while the other is at -120 volts during an alternating current cycle—a difference of 240 volts.). You can also receive a shock from electrical components that are not grounded properly. Even contact with another person who is receiving an electrical shock may cause you to be shocked.

What are the dangers of electrical shock?

Table 41.1 shows what usually happens for a range of currents (lasting one second) at typical household voltages. Longer exposure times increase the danger to the shock victim. The muscle structure of the person also makes a difference. People with less muscle tissue are typically affected at lower

Electrical And Power Outage Safety

> ### ✎ What's It Mean?
>
> <u>Circuit:</u> A complete path for the flow of current.
>
> <u>Conductor:</u> Material in which an electrical current moves easily.
>
> <u>Current:</u> The movement of electrical charge.
>
> <u>Energized (Live, "Hot"):</u> Similar terms meaning that a voltage is present that can cause a current, so there is a possibility of getting shocked.
>
> <u>Ground:</u> A physical electrical connection to the earth.
>
> <u>Neutral:</u> At ground potential (0 volts) because of a connection to ground.
>
> <u>Voltage:</u> A measure of electrical force.
>
> Source: National Institute for Occupational Safety and Health, 2002.

current levels. Even low voltages can be extremely dangerous because the degree of injury depends not only on the amount of current but also on the length of time the body is in contact with the circuit.

Sometimes high voltages lead to additional injuries. High voltages can cause violent muscular contractions. You may lose your balance and fall, which can cause injury or even death if you fall into machinery that can crush you. High voltages can also cause severe burns.

How does electricity cause burns?

The most common shock-related, nonfatal injury is a burn. Burns caused by electricity may be of three types: electrical burns, arc burns, and thermal contact burns. Electrical burns can result when a person touches electrical wiring or equipment that is used or maintained improperly. Typically, such burns occur on the hands. Electrical burns are one of the most serious injuries you can receive. They need to be given immediate attention. Additionally, clothing may catch fire and a thermal burn may result from the heat of the fire.

Arc-blasts occur when powerful, high-amperage currents arc through the air. Arcing is the luminous electrical discharge that occurs when high voltages exist across a gap between conductors and current travels through the air. This situation is often caused by equipment failure due to abuse or fatigue. Temperatures as high as 35,000° F have been reached in arc-blasts.

Table 41.1. Effects of Electrical Current* on the Body

Current	Reaction
1 milliamp	Just a faint tingle.
5 milliamps	Slight shock felt. Disturbing, but not painful. Most people can "let go." However, strong involuntary movements can cause injuries.
6–25 milliamps (women)†; 9–30 milliamps (men)	Painful shock. Muscular control is lost. This is the range where "freezing currents" start. It may not be possible to "let go."
50–150 milliamps	Extremely painful shock, respiratory arrest (breathing stops), severe muscle contractions. Flexor muscles may cause holding on; extensor muscles may cause intense pushing away. Death is possible.
1,000–4,300 milliamps (1–4.3 amps)	Ventricular fibrillation (heart pumping action not rhythmic) occurs. Muscles contract; nerve damage occurs. Death is likely.
10,000 milliamps (10 amps)	Cardiac arrest and severe burns occur. Death is probable.
15,000 milliamps (15 amps)	Lowest overcurrent at which a typical fuse or circuit breaker opens a circuit.

*Effects are for voltages less than about 600 volts. Higher voltages also cause severe burns.
†Differences in muscle and fat content affect the severity of shock.

What You Need To Know When The Power Goes Out Unexpectedly

If the power is out for less than two hours, then the food in your refrigerator and freezer will be safe to consume. While the power is out, keep the refrigerator and freezer doors closed as much as possible to keep food cold for longer. If the power is out for longer than two hours, follow the guidelines below:

Electrical And Power Outage Safety

> ### First Aid For Electrical Shock ✔ Quick Tip
>
> If you believe someone has been electrocuted take the following steps:
>
> - Look first. Don't touch. The person may still be in contact with the electrical source. Touching the person may pass the current through you.
> - Call or have someone else call 911 or emergency medical help.
> - Turn off the source of electricity if possible. If not, move the source away from you and the affected person using a nonconducting object made of cardboard, plastic or wood.
> - Once the person is free of the source of electricity, check the person's breathing and pulse. If either has stopped or seems dangerously slow or shallow, begin cardiopulmonary resuscitation (CPR) immediately.
> - If the person is faint or pale or shows other signs of shock, lay the person down with the head slightly lower than the trunk of his or her body and the legs elevated.
> - Don't touch burns, break blisters, or remove burned clothing. Electrical shock may cause burns inside the body, so be sure the person is taken to a doctor.
>
> Source: Centers for Disease Control and Prevention, January 2008.

- **For the freezer section:** A freezer that is half full will hold food safely for up to 24 hours. A full freezer will hold food safely for 48 hours. Do not open the freezer door if you can avoid it.
- **For the refrigerated section:** Pack milk, other dairy products, meat, fish, eggs, gravy, and spoilable leftovers into a cooler surrounded by ice. Inexpensive Styrofoam coolers are fine for this purpose.
- **Use a food thermometer:** Check the temperature of your food right before you cook or eat it. Throw away any food that has a temperature of more than 40 degrees Fahrenheit.

Safe Drinking Water

When power goes out, water purification systems may not be functioning fully. Safe water for drinking, cooking, and personal hygiene includes bottled, boiled, or treated water. Your state, local, or tribal health department can make specific recommendations for boiling or treating water in your area.

Extreme Heat And Cold

Heat: Be aware of yours and others' risk for heat stroke, heat exhaustion, heat cramps and fainting. To avoid heat stress, you should:

- Drink a glass of fluid every 15 to 20 minutes and at least one gallon each day. Avoid alcohol and caffeine. They both dehydrate the body.
- Wear light-colored, loose-fitting clothing.
- When indoors without air conditioning, open windows if outdoor air quality permits and use fans.
- Take frequent cool showers or baths.
- If you feel dizzy, weak, or overheated, go to a cool place. Sit or lie down, drink water, and wash your face with cool water. If you don't feel better soon, get medical help quickly.
- Work during cooler hours of the day when possible, or distribute the workload evenly throughout the day.

Heat stroke is the most serious heat illness. It happens when the body can't control its own temperature and its temperature rises rapidly. Sweating fails and the body cannot cool down. Body temperature may rise to 106° F or higher within 10 to 15 minutes. Heat stroke can cause death or permanent disability if emergency care is not given.

Warning signs of heat stroke vary but can include the following:

- Red, hot, and dry skin (no sweating)
- Rapid, strong pulse
- Throbbing headache
- Dizziness, nausea, confusion, or unconsciousness
- An extremely high body temperature (above 103° F)

Cold: Hypothermia happens when a person's core body temperature is lower than 35°C (95° F). Hypothermia has three levels: acute, subacute, or chronic.

Electrical And Power Outage Safety

- Acute hypothermia is caused by a rapid loss of body heat, usually from immersion in cold water.
- Subacute hypothermia often happens in cool outdoor weather (below 10° C or 50° F) when wind chill, wet or too little clothing, fatigue, and/or poor nutrition lower the body's ability to cope with cold.
- Chronic hypothermia happens from ongoing exposure to cold indoor temperatures (below 16° C or 60° F). The poor, the elderly, people who have hypothyroidism, people who take sedative-hypnotics, and drug and alcohol abusers are prone to chronic hypothermia, and they typically misjudge cold, move slowly, have poor nutrition, wear too little clothing, and have a poor heating system.

Causes of hypothermia include the following:

- Cold temperatures
- Improper clothing, shelter, or heating
- Wetness
- Fatigue, exhaustion
- Poor fluid intake (dehydration)
- Poor food intake
- Alcohol intake

Power Line Hazards And Cars

If a power line falls on a car, you should stay inside the vehicle. This is the safest place to stay. Warn people not to touch the car or the line. Call or ask someone to call the local utility company and emergency services.

The only circumstance in which you should consider leaving a car that is in contact with a downed power line is if the vehicle catches on fire. Open the door. Do not step out of the car. You may receive a shock. Instead, jump free of the car so that your body clears the vehicle before touching the ground. Once you clear the car, shuffle at least 50 feet away, with both feet on the ground.

As in all power line related emergencies, call for help immediately by dialing 911 or call your electric utility company's Service Center/Dispatch Office.

Do not try to help someone else from the car while you are standing on the ground.

> ✔ **Quick Tip**
> **Be Prepared For An Emergency**
>
> CDC recommends that people make an emergency plan that includes a disaster supply kit. This kit should include enough water, dried and canned food, and emergency supplies (flashlights, batteries, first-aid supplies, prescription medicines, and a digital thermometer) to last at least three days. Use battery-powered flashlights and lanterns, rather than candles, gas lanterns, or torches (to minimize the risk of fire). You can find more information on emergency plans and supply kits at http://www.ready.gov.
>
> Source: Centers for Disease Control and Prevention, January 2008.

Chapter 42

Lawn Maintenance Safety

Most people do not consider lawn maintenance to be dangerous. However, the Consumer Product Safety Commission (CPSC) reports that more than 230,000 people per year are treated for injuries from lawn and garden tools. These tools include lawn mowers, trimmers, edgers, and other power equipment. Injuries include minor to severe burns and lacerations, broken and dislocated bones, eye injuries, and loss of fingers, toes, and legs. In 2001, the CPSC reported 167 deaths associated with lawn and garden tools, more than half involving riding lawn mowers and garden tractors.

You can avoid accidents like these by making safety a regular part of lawn maintenance, particularly when using lawn mowers and other power tools.

Lawn Mower

Mowers can be walk-behind or the riding variety. Both types of mower present similar hazards to operators, bystanders, and animals that may be nearby. Rotary blades under the mower rotate at about 200 miles per hour, or 300 feet per second. Though somewhat protected by guards, all mowers are dangerous when the operator uses poor judgment or fails to follow safety procedures.

About This Chapter: "Lawn Maintenance Safety," © 2005 Texas AgriLife Extension Service (www.texasextension.tamu.edu). Reprinted with permission.

Walk-Behind Mowers

Walk-behind mowers include self-propelled and push-type mowers. These mowers are commonly used by young children because they are lightweight and easy to manipulate.

Several safety features on these mowers protect users against accidental injury. For example, all new mowers have directional flaps or shielded discharge outlets that direct grass and any other projectiles away from the operator. Since 1978, walk-behind lawn mowers have been equipped with a clutch handle or switch that stops the blade within three seconds after the operator lets go.

Walk-behind mowers can be extremely dangerous to operators and bystanders when safety guards are removed, safety shut-down devices disabled, or when the mowers are operated in a manner or environment that is unsafe. To prevent injury:

- Remove any toys, limbs, rocks, wire, or glass from the yard before mowing. Locate all sprinkler heads, exposed electrical wire or cords, tree stumps or exposed roots, and pipe.
- Keep your hands and feet away from the blade area while the mower is running.
- Never reach into the discharge chute to clear away grass or other obstructions when the blades are turning.
- Never bypass the engine kill handle or remove the shields when mowing.
- Mow back and forth along the side of a steep hill, never up and down the slope.
- Don't point the discharge chute toward bystanders.
- Wear boots or shoes with good traction to avoid slipping or falling.
- Don't allow children to operate a walk-behind mower they cannot safely control.
- To avoid spilling fuel, use a funnel when refueling a hot engine. Clean up any fuel spills immediately.
- Never smoke while servicing, operating, or refueling a mower.

Lawn Maintenance Safety

- Wear long pants, hard shoes, safety glasses, earplugs, etc., to protect yourself against flying debris and noise.

- Allow the engine to cool before returning it to a storage shed.

- Turn the power off and disconnect the spark plug wire before cleaning, inspecting, adjusting, or repairing the cutting blade.

> ♣ **It's A Fact!!**
> According to the CPSC, in 2001, more than half the 167 deaths from lawn and garden tools involved riding mowers and garden tractors.

- Don't run a gasoline-powered mower inside a storage shed—this could cause carbon monoxide poisoning.

- Never touch the spark plug with your hand or a tool when the mower is running.

- Never leave a running mower unattended, especially when children are nearby.

- Don't mow a wet lawn. Slipping on rain-soaked grass is the leading cause of foot injury by power mowers.

- Keep the cord behind you when using an electric mower. Trail it over your shoulder and always mow away from the cord.

Riding mowers save people's valuable time and energy. These small tractors are much more powerful than walk-behind mowers and move two to three times as fast. To avoid accidents on riding mowers or larger tractors, it is important to use safe driving techniques and safety devices.

Modern riding mowers come with seat safety switches that stop the cutting blades whenever the driver leaves the seat. Some riding mowers also have safety interlocks that prevent the mower from starting unless all controls are in proper position and the driver is in the seat. In addition to the safety tips listed for walk-behind mowers, take these precautions when using a riding mower:

- Don't allow extra riders.

- Test-drive the mower and become familiar with it before engaging the blades.

- Put the riding mower into neutral before starting it or turning it off.
- Watch for holes and hidden hazards.
- Don't drive too close to a creek, ditch, or any other obstruction.
- Make sure the transmission is in neutral and the mower blade disengaged before starting the engine.
- Mow up and down sloping terrain. Do not mow across a slope.
- Keep the mower in gear when going down slopes.
- Slow down when turning and when working on slopes.
- Always look behind you before backing the mower.
- Disengage the mower blade when on pavement, sidewalks, or gravel lanes.
- Don't operate a riding mower when under the influence of alcohol or other drugs that impair judgment.
- Don't let children play on the lawn where you are mowing; they could be struck by flying objects.
- Don't let children operate riding mowers until they have had proper instruction and can safely steer, brake, and adjust gears.

Power Tools

In addition to mowers, other power tools help us manicure and shape our landscapes. Electric and gas-powered weed trimmers, lawn edgers, hedge trimmers, and leaf blowers do the work that used to take days and backaches to accomplish. However, this equipment can be dangerous. In 1989, the CPSC reported that power lawn trimmers or edgers caused about 4,600 injuries requiring emergency-room treatment. About one-third of the injuries were to the eye.

Weed trimmers can throw stones, sticks, and other objects at high speeds. Lawn edgers with metal blades can cut through underground objects, splinter concrete, or cause sparks. Hedge trimmers are sometimes heavy, and fatigue can cause cutting accidents. Leaf blowers are loud and can produce air gusts in excess of 200 miles per hour that can lift small rocks and other objects into the air. Users must take special care to prevent these accidents with these tools.

Lawn Maintenance Safety

Weed Trimmers

- Before trimming, remove glass, limbs, rocks, and trash that could become projectiles.

- Watch for exposed electrical wires, communication lines, and extension cords to avoid damaging them with the trimmer string.

- Don't remove protective guards and string guides.

- Monitor the string length. Automatic-feed and bump-feed trimmers may release more string than you think and cause the string to strike you unexpectedly.

- Make sure all children and bystanders are out of the way before you begin trimming.

- Protect yourself with long pants, long-sleeve shirts, gloves, hard boots, goggles or safety glasses, and earplugs.

- With electric trimmers, inspect all extension cords for cuts, nicks, or scrapes. Exposed wires are an electrical hazard. Replace damaged cords immediately.

- Don't operate electric trimmers around water puddles or in wet conditions.

- Unplug electric trimmers and turn off gas-powered trimmers before inspecting, cleaning, adjusting, or replacing the string.

- Never leave an electric trimmer plugged in or a gas-powered trimmer running while unattended.

- Before refueling, place the gas-powered trimmer on the ground and allow the engine to cool.

Lawn Edgers

- Make sure all children and bystanders are at a safe distance before starting the edger.

- Don't start an edger if the blade is touching the ground. It could move unpredictably and injure your feet or legs.

- Watch out for exposed electrical wires, communication lines, and extension cords that could be struck by the edger.
- Wear goggles or safety glasses to guard against flying objects.
- Don't remove the protective guards or shields.
- Operate the edger at full blade speed.
- When edging along roadways, stay as close to the curb as possible to avoid being hit by passing vehicles.
- Never leave an electric- or gas-powered edger plugged in or running while unattended.
- Unplug or turn off an electric or gas-powered edger before inspecting, cleaning, adjusting, or replacing the blade.

Hedge Trimmers

- Wear gloves, goggles or safety glasses, and ear plugs.
- Make sure all screws, blades, or chains are secure. Vibrating equipment can cause the screws to loosen.
- Keep extension cords clear of blades.
- Disconnect extension cords and shut down hedge trimmers before inspecting, cleaning, adjusting, or replacing the blades.
- Do not leave hedge trimmers unattended; they have sharp blades and can injure children and others.
- Never use an electric hedge trimmer overhead. If the trimmer becomes lodged, disconnect the power before trying to dislodge it.

Leaf Blowers

- Don't use the blower to clean debris off of yourself.
- Be aware of pedestrians and others in the area. Don't direct the blower toward bystanders.
- Wear goggles or safety glasses and earplugs.

Lawn Maintenance Safety

- With electric blowers, inspect all extension cords for cuts, nicks, scrapes, or exposed wire that could pose an electrical hazard. Replace damaged cords immediately.
- Don't operate electric blowers around water puddles or when conditions are wet.

Lawn And Garden Chemicals

People and landscape maintenance companies periodically apply natural and synthetic insecticides, herbicides, and fungicides to control a variety of insects, weeds, and plant diseases. If you use a lawn and garden chemical, read the product label carefully to determine its toxicity to humans, animals, and the environment. The label will give the recommended application rate and instructions, and will list any protective clothing or equipment required. Use only the amount of chemical specified.

Consider the potential effects on the environment and beneficial insects in your landscape when selecting lawn and garden chemicals. For example, instead of using a general-purpose pesticide, use a product that treats only the specific problem.

Other precautions include:

- Keep children and animals away from the application area. Follow label directions regarding re-entry into the treated area.
- Protect your skin, eyes, and nose during and after application.
- Close all doors and windows to the house.
- Remove animal water and food containers. Protect bird baths and fish ponds from chemical exposure.
- Avoid over-irrigating treatment area because pesticides may be washed away or become concentrated in standing water puddles.
- Use only the recommended amount. Excess application will not do a better job.
- After application, store extra chemicals out of reach of children and pets.

- Never store lawn and garden chemicals with or near food, animal feeds, or medical supplies.

Taking precautions when using and maintaining lawn equipment and chemicals can help you avoid accidents associated with lawn maintenance.

✔ **Quick Tip**
Keep chemicals locked in a well-ventilated storage area, where temperatures stay above freezing and less than 90 degrees.

Chapter 43

What Working Teens Need To Know About Safety

Could I get hurt or sick on the job?

Every year about 70 teens die from work injuries in the United States. Another 70,000 get hurt badly enough that they go to a hospital emergency room.

Why do injuries like these occur? Teens are often injured on the job due to unsafe equipment, stressful conditions, and speed-up. Also teens may not receive adequate safety training and supervision. As a teen, one is much more likely to be injured when working on jobs that they are not allowed to do by law.

What are my rights on the job?

By law, your employer must provide the following:

- A safe and healthful workplace

- Safety and health training, in many situations, including providing information on chemicals that could be harmful to your health

- For many jobs, payment for medical care if you get hurt or sick because of your job. You may also be entitled to lost wages.

About This Chapter: From "Are You A Working Teen?" National Institute for Occupational Safety and Health, 1997; available online at http://www.cdc.gov/niosh/adoldoc.html, accessed February 2008.

- At least the Federal minimum wage to most teens after their first 90 days on the job. Many states have minimum wages which may be higher than the Federal wage, and lower wages may be allowed when workers receive tips from customers. (Call your state Department of Labor listed in the blue pages of your phone book for information on minimum wages in your state).

You also have a right to do these things:

- Report safety problems to Occupational Safety and Health Administration (OSHA)
- Work without racial or sexual harassment
- Refuse to work if the job is immediately dangerous to your life or health
- Join or organize a union

What hazards should I watch out for?

Janitor/Clean-Up
- Toxic chemicals in cleaning products
- Blood on discarded needles

Food Service
- Slippery floors
- Hot cooking equipment
- Sharp objects

Retail/Sales
- Violent crimes
- Heavy lifting

Office/Clerical
- Stress
- Harassment
- Poor computer work station design

♣ It's A Fact!! Jobs Teens Can Do

- **When you are 13 or younger:** You can babysit, deliver newspapers, or work as an actor or performer.
- **When you turn 14:** You can work in an office, grocery store, retail store, restaurant, movie theater, or amusement park.
- **When you turn 16:** You can work in any job that is not hazardous.

Youth cannot work in mining, logging, meatpacking, roofing, excavation, or demolition. You cannot drive a car or forklift. You cannot work with saws, explosives, radioactive materials, or most power-driven machines.

Source: "Youth Rules," U.S. Department of Labor, undated; accessed February 2008.

What Working Teens Need To Know About Safety

Is it OK to do any kind of work?

NO. There are laws that protect teens from doing dangerous work. No worker under 18 may do the following:

- Drive a motor vehicle as a regular part of the job or operate a forklift at any time
- Operate many types of powered equipment like a circular saw, box crusher, meat slicer, or bakery machine
- Work in wrecking, demolition, excavation, or roofing
- Work in mining, logging, or a sawmill
- Work in meat-packing or slaughtering
- Work where there is exposure to radiation
- Work where explosives are manufactured or stored

Also, no one 14 or 15 years old may do these jobs:

- Bake or cook on the job (except at a serving counter)
- Operate power-driven machinery, except certain types which pose little hazard such as those used in offices
- Work on a ladder or scaffold

♣ It's A Fact!!
Work On The Farm

- **Ages 12 or 13:** Can be employed in non-hazardous jobs, outside school hours on farms that also employ the youth's parent(s) or with written parental consent.
- **Ages 14 or 15:** Can be employed in non-hazardous jobs, outside school hours.
- **Age 16 or Older:** Can be employed in any farm job, hazardous or not, at any time.

Source: "Youth Rules (Farm)," U.S. Department of Labor, undated; accessed February 2008.

> ♣ **It's A Fact!!**
>
> **Work On The Farm**
>
> Youths of any age may work at any time in any job on a farm owned or operated by their parents or persons standing in place of their parents.
>
> There are 11 specific hazardous occupations in agriculture that may only be performed by hired farmworkers who are at least 16 years of age. Most involve work with machinery or handling toxic or explosive materials. Some limited exemptions exist that permit 14- and 15-year-olds to perform these otherwise prohibited tasks if they are enrolled in a vocational agriculture program or have received appropriate training.
>
> Source: "Youth Rules (Farm)," U.S. Department of Labor, undated; accessed February 2008.

- Work in warehouses
- Work in construction, building, or manufacturing
- Load or unload a truck, railroad car, or conveyor

Are there other things I can't do?

YES. There are many other restrictions regarding the type of work you can and cannot do.

If you are under 14, there are even stricter laws to protect your health and safety. States have their own child labor laws which may be stricter than the federal laws.

Check with your school counselor, job placement coordinator, or state Department of Labor to make sure the job you are doing is allowed.

What are my safety responsibilities on the job?

To work safely you should observe these guidelines:

- Follow all safety rules and instructions.
- Use safety equipment and protective clothing when needed.
- Look out for co-workers.

What Working Teens Need To Know About Safety

- Keep work areas clean and neat.
- Know what to do in an emergency.
- Report any health and safety hazard to your supervisor.

Should I be working this late or this long?

Federal child labor laws protect younger teens from working too long, too late, or too early. Some states have laws on the hours that older teens may work.

Work Hours For Ages 14 And 15

- Work Hours not before 7 a.m. or after 7 p.m. between Labor Day and June 1
- Not during school hours
- 7 a.m.–9 p.m. between June 1 and Labor Day
- Maximum hours when school is in session: 18 hours a week, but not over three hours a day on school days or eight hours a day Saturday, Sunday, and holidays
- Maximum hours when school is not in session: 40 hours a week and eight hours a day

What if I need help?

- Talk to your boss about the problem.
- Talk to your parents or teachers.
- For a Hazard Alert on preventing injuries and deaths of adolescent workers or for information on specific workplace hazards, contact NIOSH at

---

♣ It's A Fact!!
Work Hours For Teens

If you are 14 or 15, you can work:

- Outside school hours
- After 7 a.m. and until 7 p.m. during the school year (9 p.m. in the summer)
- 3 hours on a school day
- 18 hours in a school week
- 8 hours on a non-school day
- 40 hours in non-school week

If you are 16 or older, you can work any hours.

Different rules apply to farms, and state laws may have stricter rules.

Source: "Youth Rules," U.S. Department of Labor, undated; accessed February 2008.

800-35-NIOSH (800-356-4674) and ask for Report #95-125 or visit the NIOSH homepage at http://www.cdc.gov/niosh/homepage.html.

- For more information on working safe, visit the Department of Labor website at http://www.dol.gov or call your local Wage and Hour Office (under Department of Labor in the blue pages of your local telephone book).

- If necessary contact one of these government agencies. (Phone numbers can be found under Department of Labor in the blue pages of your local telephone book).

  - OSHA—to make a health or safety complaint.
  - Wage and Hour—to make a complaint about wages, work hours, or illegal work by youth less than 18 years of age.
  - Equal Employment Opportunities Commission—to make a complaint about sexual harassment or discrimination.

You have a right to speak up. It is illegal for your employer to fire or punish you for reporting a workplace problem.

Part Five
Outdoor And Recreation Safety

Chapter 44

Sports And Exercise Safety

Lots of teens are injured while playing sports—but getting hurt doesn't have to happen. A few sports injury prevention steps can help to keep everyone in the game. Read on to learn the basics of sports and exercise safety.

Essential Equipment

Did you know that playing tennis with a badly strung (too loose or too tight) racquet while wearing worn-out shoes can be just as dangerous as playing football without shoulder pads? Using the wrong—or improperly fitted—equipment is a major reason why teens get injured.

The equipment you wear while participating in sports and other activities is key to preventing injuries. Start with helmets: They are important for sports such as football, hockey, baseball, softball, biking, skateboarding, in-line skating, skiing, and snowboarding—to name just a few.

- Always wear a helmet made for the sport you're playing.
- When choosing a bike helmet, look for a sticker that says the helmet meets the safety standard set by the Consumer Product Safety

---

About This Chapter: "Sports and Exercise Safety," December 2004, reprinted with permission from www.kidshealth.org. Copyright © 2004 The Nemours Foundation. This information was provided by KidsHealth, one of the largest resources online for medically reviewed health information written for parents, kids, and teens. For more articles like this one, visit www.KidsHealth.org, or www.TeensHealth.org.

Commission (CPSC), a part of the United States government that creates safety standards for bike helmets and other safety equipment.

- If you use a multi-sport helmet for in-line skating and skateboarding, it is not considered safe for bicycle riding unless it has the CPSC sticker.
- Any helmet should fit snugly but comfortably on your head and shouldn't tilt backward or forward.

Eye protection also is a must for many sports:

- The most protective eye gear is made from a plastic called polycarbonate and has been tested especially for sports use.
- Face masks or polycarbonate guards or shields that attach to a helmet are worn in sports such as football, ice hockey, and softball and baseball when batting.
- Goggles are often worn for soccer, basketball, racquet sports, snowboarding, street hockey, and baseball and softball when fielding.
- If you wear glasses, you'll probably need prescription polycarbonate goggles—don't just wear your regular glasses when you're on the court or field.
- All eye protection should fit securely and have cushions above your eyebrows and over your nose.

Mouth guards can protect your mouth, teeth, and tongue:

- You should wear a mouth guard if you play a contact sport or other sport where head injury is a risk, such as football, basketball, hockey, volleyball, martial arts, boxing, or wrestling.
- Mouth guards can be fitted for your mouth by a dentist or purchased at sports stores.
- If you wear a retainer, always take it out before you start to exercise, practice, or play.

Wrist, knee, and elbow guards are important gear, too:

- If you in-line skate, skateboard, or ride a scooter, you should wear guards.

Sports And Exercise Safety

- Elbow and wrist guards can prevent arm and wrist fractures, and knee guards can shield your knees from cuts and breaks.

If you play certain sports, especially contact sports, pads are essential:

- All kinds of sports, from hockey to in-line skating, use pads. There are shin, knee, elbow, wrist, chest, shoulder, hip, and thigh pads.
- Check with your coach or doctor to find out what kinds of pads you might need for your sport.

Some guys may also need to wear a protective cup:

- Guys who play hockey, football, basketball, baseball, soccer, and other contact sports should use a cup.
- For non-contact sports that involve running, guys should wear an athletic supporter.
- If you're unsure, ask your coach, athletic trainer, or parent if you need a cup for your sport.

And last but not least, the right footwear can keep you from tripping and falling:

- You know that sports like football, baseball, softball, and soccer require cleats. But you may not realize that sports like skateboarding and biking need special types of shoes, too. Ask your coach or doctor what shoes are best for your sport.
- Replace shoes and cleats that have worn out or are no longer supportive.

Warm Up To Keep Your Game Up

Don't rush into any sport or exercise without warming up first—muscles that haven't been properly prepared tend to be injured more

> ♣ **It's A Fact!!**
> Not only is the right kind of equipment important, so is the right fit. If you don't know if your equipment fits properly, check with a coach, gym teacher, athletic trainer, or parent to make sure you have the right size and that you're wearing it correctly. Many sporting goods stores can also help you find the right fit. The bottom line: Wearing the right equipment with the right fit dramatically decreases your chances of getting hurt.

easily. Start out with some light cardiovascular activities, such as easy jogging, jumping jacks, or brisk walking, just to get your muscles going. Follow your brief warm-up with some stretches. (Stretching works best after a warm-up because your tissues are more elastic and flexible due to the increase in heat and blood flow to the muscles).

In addition to warm-ups and stretches, practice sessions are also an excellent preparation for most sports or activities. If you belong to a team, attend as many team practices and games as possible. This will put you in top physical condition and help you and your teammates work together—and knowing how your teammates play will help prevent injuries.

Even if you don't belong to a team, you can use regular workouts and practices to enhance your performance and lessen the chance of injuries. Remember, if a tool isn't used, it gets rusty, so keep yourself in top shape with regular practice. For instance, try doing tennis drills or practicing your serve before starting a set. Shoot some baskets or play a quick game of one-on-one with a friend. Practice gets your brain and body to work together while improving your performance.

Although you should practice regularly, don't overdo it. Sudden increases in training frequency, duration, or intensity might produce better performance at first but can lead to injuries later. Your doctor or coach can help you develop a training and conditioning program that's appropriate for your age and level of development.

Staying Off The Court When You're Hurt

If you've been injured and you try to come back too soon, you run the great risk of re-injuring yourself—maybe even more seriously than before. Don't let anyone—including yourself, your parents, your friends, or even your coach—pressure you into playing before your body is fully healed. Your doctor, coach, or trainer will give you specific advice on when you should return to your sport or activity.

Taking time to heal is particularly important if you've had a concussion. Lots of athletes try to come back too quickly after getting a concussion—because they can't see an injury, they think they're okay to play. But jumping back into the game too soon puts a player at greater risk for another concussion—and that can lead to a dangerous brain injury. So always get clearance from your doctor to play again if you've had a concussion.

Many athletes use pain relievers to avoid pain. If you feel persistent pain, don't use pain relievers to mask it, though. Taking large amounts of pain relievers—or, worse yet, taking pain relievers for a long time in order to play—can be dangerous. Pain is the body's way of signaling it's not happy with what you're doing. If you have a lot of pain, seek treatment so you can resolve what's causing it.

The same advice goes for a cold or flu virus—don't play if you're sick. You won't be able to concentrate if your head is stuffed up and your nose is running faster than you are, and your lack of concentration can put you at risk for injury. It's better to wait until you feel better, so you can have a safe season.

> ♣ **It's A Fact!!**
> Be sure to seek medical treatment whenever you experience:
> - moderate to severe pain;
> - pain that interferes with daily activity or sleep;
> - swelling of the injured area;
> - an inability to perform normal activities.

The Rules Of The Game

Rules and regulations usually exist for a good reason—to keep you and your teammates in the game and to avoid injuries. Do yourself a favor and learn the rules thoroughly—and then follow them. Rules aren't restrictions. They're designed to promote safety so that everyone can enjoy the game. For example, a late hit in football after the referee's whistle has blown leads to a pretty big penalty. This rule is important because a player could be seriously injured if he or she is not expecting a tackle after play has stopped.

Sometimes rules may not be directly related to a sport or activity but need to be followed anyway. For instance, if you're in-line skating, skateboarding, or riding a bike, pay strict attention to all traffic laws, especially when riding on busy public streets.

Proper techniques also promote safety. This goes for any sport, from motor racing to baseball. Baseball players know not to spike the opposing player who's covering the bag, even when sliding hard into second base. And when two tennis players rush the net, an expertly angled volley is the correct shot—not a hard smash socked directly at an opponent's face.

Another example of a safe technique occurs in weight lifting. Weightlifters should take a breath between each repetition. Exhale on the pushing phase of a lift. So if you're doing a bench press, let the bar come down to your chest, and if you're pushing up, breathe out. Holding your breath can raise your blood pressure, and if you're pressing a lot of weight this can lead to a blackout or fainting spell.

So whether you're following rules, regulations, or proper techniques, remember that they aren't there to restrict you—they're there to keep you safe and injury free.

Chapter 45

Safe Bicycling

Bicycling is one of the most popular ways to get around, whether for recreation, sport or transportation. An estimated 57 million Americans ride bikes ranging from high performance, 18-speed, touring models, to "dirt bikes" equipped with balloon tires—and dozens of variations in between.

With millions of cyclists on the roads—the same roads occupied by millions of motor vehicles that are larger, heavier, and faster than bikes—the National Safety Council believes that defensive driving applies to people who pedal with their feet to travel, as well as to those who push on the gas pedal. Because about 900 bicyclists were killed and some 70,000 suffered disabling injuries (1999 statistics), it is clear that taking precautions in traffic and wearing protective equipment are a cyclist's best shields against unintentional injuries.

The Council offers the following tips for safe and enjoyable bicycling:

- Obey traffic rules. Get acquainted with ordinances. Cyclists must follow the same rules as motorists.

- Know your bike's capabilities. Remember that bicycles differ from motor vehicles; they're smaller and can't move as fast. But, they can

---

About This Chapter: This chapter begins with "Safe Bicycling," © 2004 National Safety Council (www.nsc.org). Reprinted with permission. Additional information is from "Hard Facts about Helmets," BAM! (Body and Mind), Centers for Disease Control and Prevention (CDC), 2002.

change direction more easily, stop faster, and move through smaller spaces.

- Ride in single file with traffic, not against it. Bicycling two abreast can be dangerous. Bicyclists should stay as far right on the pavement as possible, watching for opening car doors, sewer gratings, soft shoulders, broken glass, and other debris. Remember to keep a safe distance from the vehicle ahead.

- Make safe turns and cross intersections with care. Signal turns half a block before the intersection, using the correct hand signals (left arm straight out for left turn; forearm up for right turn). When traffic is heavy and the cyclist has to turn left, it is best to dismount and walk the bicycle across both streets at the crosswalks.

- Never hitch on cars. A sudden stop or turn could send the cyclist flying into the path of another vehicle.

- Before riding into traffic: stop, look left, right, left again, and over your shoulder.

- Always be seen. During the day, cyclists should wear bright clothing. Nighttime cycling is not advised, but if riding at night is necessary, retroreflective clothing, designed to bounce back motorists' headlight beams, will make cyclists more visible.

- Make sure the bicycle has the right safety equipment: a red rear reflector; a white front reflector; a red or colorless spoke reflector on the rear wheel; an amber or colorless reflector on the front wheel; pedal reflectors; a horn or bell; and a rear view mirror. A bright headlight is recommended for night riding.

- Wear a helmet. Head injuries cause about 85 percent of all bicycling fatalities. The Council strongly urges all cyclists to wear helmets. The first body part to fly forward in a collision is usually the head, and with nothing but skin and bone to protect the brain from injury, the results can be disastrous.

- In March 1999, the U.S. Consumer Product Safety Commission (CPSC) issued a uniform, mandatory federal safety standard for all bike helmets. All helmets manufactured or imported for sale in the U.S. must carry a label or sticker stating that they meet the requirements of the new standard. Cyclists who currently have a helmet that meets the American Society for Testing and Material (ASTM), American National Standards Institute (ANSI), or Snell standards do not need to rush out to buy a new one; these helmets provide adequate protection. However, when it's time to replace a helmet because it has been outgrown or damaged in a crash, buying a helmet that meets the CPSC standard is recommended. The helmet should fit securely and should be worn low and near the eyebrows—not back on the forehead.

A properly designed helmet has four characteristics:

1. A stiff outer shell designed to distribute impact forces and protect against sharp objects;

2. An energy-absorbing liner at least one-half inch thick;

3. Chin strap and fastener to keep the helmet in place; and,

4. It should be lightweight, cool in hot weather, and fit comfortably.

There is no limit to the fun and healthful exercise gained from bicycling. Being careful, always, will give riders safer trips and greater peace of mind.

Hard Facts About Helmets

If you like recreational activities that involve wheels, concrete, or asphalt, then protect your brain by wearing a helmet. Helmets with a CPSC approval are good for biking and in-line skating and are available in most sporting goods stores. "Multi-sport" helmets with a Snell B-95 approval are designed for skateboarding, roller-skating, and riding scooters as well as biking and in-line skating. Snell B-95 rated helmets provide more protection but you may have to check out more stores to find one.

Your helmet should sit flat on your head—make sure it is level and is not tilted back or forward. The front of the helmet should sit low—about two finger widths above your eyebrows to protect your forehead. The straps on each side of your head should form a "Y" over your ears, with one part of the

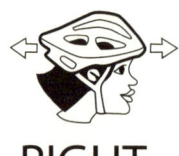

RIGHT

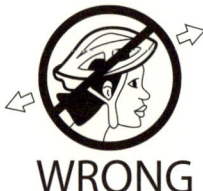

WRONG

Figure 45.1. The proper way to wear a bicycle helmet (Source: CDC, 2002).

strap in front of your ear, and one behind—just below your earlobes. If the helmet leans forward, adjust the rear straps. If it tilts backward, tighten the front straps. Buckle the chinstrap securely at your throat so that the helmet feels snug on your head and does not move up and down or from side to side.

> ♣ **It's A Fact!!**
>
> ### Helmets...Fact Or Fiction?
>
> **Fiction:** Helmets aren't cool.
>
> **Fact:** Who says helmets can't be cool? If you're shopping for a helmet, there are lots of options, so you can pick out your favorite color. Or decorate your helmet with stickers and reflectors to show your personal style. Helmets are designed to help prevent injuries to your head, 'cause a serious fall or crash can cause permanent brain damage or death. And that's definitely not cool.
>
> **Fiction:** Helmets just aren't comfortable.
>
> **Fact:** Today's helmets are lightweight, well ventilated, and have lots of padding. Try on your helmet to make sure it fits properly and comfortably on your head before you buy it.
>
> **Fiction:** Really good riders don't need to wear helmets.
>
> **Fact:** Bike crashes or collisions can happen at any time. Even professional bike racers get in serious wrecks. In three out of four bike crashes, bikers usually get some sort of injury to their head.
>
> Source: CDC, 2002.

Chapter 46

Water Sports And Boating

H2O Smarts

What do surfing, fishing, water skiing, and swimming have in common? They are all lots of fun...and they all take place in, on, or around the water. Water activities are a great way to stay cool and have a good time with your friends or your family. Take along these tips—and your common sense—to get wet, make waves, and have a blast.

Top Ten Tips

- Do learn to swim. If you like to have a good time doing water activities, being a strong swimmer is a must.

- Do take a friend along. Even though you may be a good swimmer, you never know when you may need help. Having friends around is safer and just more fun.

- Do know your limits. Watch out for the "toos"—too tired, too cold, too far from safety, too much sun, too much hard activity.

- Do swim in supervised (watched) areas only, and follow all signs and warnings.

About This Chapter: This chapter includes "H2O Smarts," BAM! (Body and Mind), Centers for Disease Control and Prevention, 2002; "Life Jacket Wear," U.S. Coast Guard (USCG), 2005; and "Beware Boat Propellers," USCG, undated.

- Do wear a life jacket when boating, jet skiing, water skiing, rafting, or fishing.
- Do stay alert to currents. They can change quickly. If you get caught in a strong current, don't fight it. Swim parallel to the shore until you have passed through it. Near piers, jetties (lines of big rocks), small dams, and docks, the current gets unpredictable and could knock you around. If you find it hard to move around, head to shore. Learn to recognize and watch for dangerous waves and signs of rip currents—water that is a weird color, really choppy, foamy, or filled with pieces of stuff.
- Do keep an eye on the weather. If you spot bad weather (dark clouds, lighting), pack up and take the fun inside.
- Don't mess around in the water. Pushing or dunking your friends can get easily out of hand.
- Don't dive into shallow water. If you don't know how deep the water is, don't dive.
- Don't float where you can't swim. Keep checking to see if the water is too deep, or if you are too far away from the shore or the poolside.

Watch Out For Mother Nature

Even if you are an expert, things that you can't control can get you into trouble.

Look out for signs warning you that the water is not clean, because polluted water could make you sick. (And even if it is clean, try not to swallow it. Yuck.)

It's also smart to keep clear of objects in the water like water plants and animals. They can cause problems for you so, if you see them—go the other way. (You've heard about what jellyfish and snapping turtles can do, right?)

Finally, if you're outside, you need to guard against the sun. Those burning rays reflect off the water and sand onto you…and they can really spoil the fun. So, rub on some sunscreen to get sun proof.

The Deal On Water Parks

If you've ever been to a water park, you know that they are so much fun. Read these Body and Mind (BAM!) need-to-knows for having a great time on ride after ride:

Water Sports And Boating

> ♣ **It's A Fact!!**
>
> ### Water Wisdom
>
> *Icy*
>
> If the water's cold, a wetsuit can be your best friend. Wearing it will make you feel more comfortable, and you'll keep your body temp from dropping to the danger zone.
>
> *Floaters Vs. PFDs*
>
> Q: Can blow-up objects such as rafts work like life preservers?
>
> A: Nope. Although they float, they won't do the trick.
>
> Source: BAM! (Body and Mind), Centers for Disease Control and Prevention, 2002.

Read all the signs before going on a ride. Make sure you are tall enough and old enough. Ask questions if you are not sure about how you're supposed to go on the ride. (On most water slides, you should go down face up, arms crossed behind your head, and feet first with your ankles crossed.)

When you go from ride to ride, don't run. It's slippery.

Bumping into others on a slide can hurt. That's why no "chains" of people are allowed on water rides. So, count five seconds after the rider ahead of you has gone before you take your turn.

Wear a life preserver—the park supplies it for a reason.

The Deal On Boating And Jet Skiing

Skimming over the water is a great ride. You probably aren't driving a boat or jet ski yourself just yet, but they are lots of fun to ride with an adult. (Remember, they like to have fun too.) You and your parents can check the state rules for how old you have to be, and cruise through this boating site.

Stay alert. When you're riding, keep a lookout for other boats, jet skiers, water skiers, divers, and swimmers. Who has the right-of-way? Generally, drivers should keep to their right when they are passing other boats—just like you do when you are walking in the hall at school.

Always ride at a speed that will let you stay in control so you can stop or go another way if you need to. It's also not a good idea to jump wakes (tracks in the water left by other boats or jet skis) or speed through choppy water, because it's easy to loose control.

Do not ride with a driver who has been drinking alcohol.

Make sure you know and practice what to do if someone falls out of the boat.

Some people teak surf (hold on to the back of the boat and then let go to ride the wave that the boat makes), but you shouldn't copy them. Teak surfers get too close to the boat, don't wear life jackets, and breathe exhaust fumes (chemicals) that the boat makes. Sounds like a bad idea to us.

Life Jacket Wear

The U.S. Coast Guard estimates that life jackets could have saved the lives of over 80 percent of boating fatality victims.

As a boat operator, you're in command of the safety of your passengers. But accidents can, and do happen with terrifying speed on the water. There's rarely time to reach stowed life jackets.

The U.S. Coast Guard challenges you and your passengers to wear your life jacket all the time while underway.

New Life Jackets Are Attractive And Easy To Wear

Boaters enjoy the feel of sun and spray. So it's tempting to boat without wearing a life jacket—especially on nice days. But modern life jackets are available in a wide variety of shapes, colors, and sizes. Many are thin and flexible. Some are built right into fishing vests or hunter coats.

> ♣ **It's A Fact!!**
> **Lifeline**
>
> If you see someone struggling in the water, go get help. You can also throw out a life preserver or other object that floats, but do not jump in yourself.
>
> If you jump in without anyone else around, who will help save you if there is a problem? There are a whole lot of ways to have a great time in the water.
>
> Source: BAM! (Body and Mind), Centers for Disease Control and Prevention, 2002.

Water Sports And Boating

Others are inflatable—as compact as a scarf or fanny pack until they hit water, when they automatically fill with air.

There's no excuse not to wear a life jacket on the water.

Things To Know

- Certain life jackets are designed to keep your head above water and help you remain in a position which permits proper breathing.
- To meet U.S. Coast Guard requirements, a boat must have a U.S. Coast Guard-approved Type I, II, III, or V life jacket for each person aboard. Boats 16 feet and over must have at least one Type IV throwable device as well.
- All states have regulations regarding life jacket wear by children.
- Adult-sized life jackets will not work for children. Special life jackets are available. To work correctly, a life jacket must be worn, fit snugly, and not allow the child's chin or ears to slip through.
- Life jackets should be tested for wear and buoyancy at least once each year. Waterlogged, faded, or leaky jackets should be discarded.
- Life jackets must be properly stowed.
- A life jacket—especially a snug-fitting flotation coat or deck-suit style—can help you survive in cold water.

How Do Life Jackets Save Lives?

- When capsized in rough water.
- When sinking in unexpectedly heavy sea conditions.
- When thrown from the boat as a result of a collision.
- When injured by rocks or submerged objects.
- When unconscious from carbon monoxide fumes.
- When tossed into freezing water.
- When thrown off balance while fishing.
- When unable to swim because of heavy or waterlogged clothing.

Understand The Danger Of Propeller Strikes

A typical three-blade propeller running at 3,200 rpm can inflict 160 impacts in one second. A typical recreational propeller can travel from head to toe on an average person in less than one tenth of a second. Most propeller accidents CAN be prevented.

What Can You Do?

- Wear your engine cut-off switch lanyard and your life jacket at ALL times. If the lanyard is removed from the switch, the engine will shut off.
- Assign a passenger to keep watch around the propeller area of your boat when people are in the water.
- Consider purchasing propeller safety devices for your boat.

Safety Tips

- Before starting your boat, walk to the stern and look in the water to make certain there is no one near your propeller (people near propeller may not be visible from helm).
- Never allow passengers to board or exit your boat from the water when engines are on—or idling (your propeller may continue to spin).
- Educate passengers about the location and danger of the propellers.
- Call attention to and discuss any propeller warning labels around your boat.
- Be especially alert when operating in congested areas and never enter swimming zones.
- Take extra precautions near boats that are towing skiers or tubers.
- Never permit passengers to ride on the bow, gunwale, transom, seatbacks, or other locations where they might fall overboard.
- Children should be watched carefully while onboard.
- Establish clear rules for swim platform use, boarding ladders, and seating (if possible, passengers should remain seated at all times).

Water Sports And Boating

- If someone falls overboard, stop. Then slowly turn the boat around, and keep the person in sight as you approach. Assign a passenger to continuously monitor the person in the water. Turn your engine off first and then bring the person to safety.

- Never reverse your boat to pick someone up out of the water. Go around again.

♣ It's A Fact!!

Safety Devices

A variety of safety devices are available to help prevent propeller strikes:

- Wireless cut-off switches
- Propeller guards
- Ringed propellers
- Propulsion alternatives
- Interlocks
- Sensors
- Anti-feedback steering

Source: "Understand the Danger of Propeller Strikes," USCG.

Chapter 47

All-Terrain Vehicles (ATVs)

All-Terrain Vehicle (ATV) Safety

ATVs have become popular for work and recreation on many farms and ranches. Unfortunately, reported cases of serious injury and death have increased along with their increased use. Most of these injuries and deaths can be attributed to improper use of ATVs. Make ATV safety a priority on your farm or ranch.

- An ATV is not a toy. Children should not be permitted to operate ATVs without specialized training and then they should be allowed to only operate an ATV of an appropriate size. Contact the ATV Safety Institute (http://www.atvsafety.org) to enroll in a course.

- ATVs with an engine size of 70 cc to 90 cc should be operated by people at least 12 years of age.

- ATVs with an engine size of greater than 90 cc should only be operated by people at least 16 years of age.

- Wear appropriate riding gear: Department of Transportation (DOT)-, Snell-, American National Standards Institute (ANSI)-approved helmet, goggles, gloves, over-the-ankle boots, long-sleeve shirt, and long pants.

About This Chapter: This chapter begins with "All-Terrain Vehicle (ATV) Safety," © 2004 National Safety Council (www.nsc.org). Reprinted with permission. Additional text from Safe Kids Worldwide is cited separately within the chapter.

- Read owners manuals carefully.
- ATVs are not made for multiple riders. Never carry anyone else on the ATV.
- Any added attachments affect the stability, operating, and braking of the ATV.
- Just because an attachment is available doesn't mean that it can be used without increasing your risk of being injured.
- Do not operate the ATV on streets, highways, or paved roads.

Inspection

- Are tires and wheels in good condition?
- Are controls and cable operational?
- Does the chain have proper slack and is it lubricated?
- Is riding gear (including a helmet) available and worn?

No Children Under 16 On ATVs

"Safety Experts Remind Parents: No Children Under 16 on ATVs," © 2007 Safe Kids Worldwide. Reprinted with permission.

While wearing a helmet can reduce the risk of head injuries, there are no safety devices that adequately protect against other injuries commonly sustained while riding ATVs. Accordingly, Safe Kids Worldwide recommends that no children under age 16 be allowed to ride an ATV under any circumstances.

Compared to a bike crash, an ATV crash is six times as likely to send a child to the hospital and 12 times as likely to kill a child. A child riding an ATV is four times as likely to be seriously injured as a rider over age 16.

ATV rollovers, collisions, and ejections can cause instantly fatal head injuries as well as serious nonfatal injuries to the head, spinal cord, and abdomen. ATVs are inherently difficult to operate, and children do not have the cognitive and physical abilities to drive or ride these vehicles safely. A child who is not old enough to drive a car on a paved road with traffic control devices is certainly not old enough to drive a powerful open-seat vehicle at speeds up to 70 miles per hour over dirt trails.

All-Terrain Vehicles (ATVs)

Previous efforts to make ATVs safer for kids have proved inadequate. Government efforts and the voluntary standards observed by the industry have not kept children out of the emergency room. On the contrary, the number of kids getting seriously injured on ATVs every year is increasing.

In 1998, the U.S. Consumer Product Safety Commission banned the manufacture of three-wheeled ATVs, mandated warning labels, and set standards for the engine size of ATVs intended for children. Ten years later, the ATV industry adopted policies restricting the sale of adult-sized ATVs (with engines bigger than 90 cc) for use by children under age 16.

The number of ATV-related injuries per year doubled between 1993 and 2001, and the injury and death rates are highest among riders under 16. In 2003, children accounted for nearly one third of all ATV-related injuries.

After extensive review of the data, Safe Kids Worldwide concludes that there is simply no way to make ATV riding a safe activity for children.

♣ **It's A Fact!!**
All-terrain vehicles are involved in approximately 38,000 injuries and 100 deaths to children ages 16 and under each year.

Source: © 2007 Safe Kids Worldwide.

Chapter 48

Snowmobile Safety

Across a special part of North America, summer weather is uncertain but winter always brings snow. More than 10 million people look forward to that blanket of white and the pleasures of enjoying the outdoors on snowmobiles.

Many things make snowmobiling fun: the breathtaking beauty of a snow-filled woods, field, or mountain; the precision performance of a well-designed machine; the satisfaction of traversing the winter landscape with friends and family.

Yes, snowmobilers savor the winter world, and that calls for extra responsibility. Training, experience and awareness are all traits of the accomplished snowmobiler. You are the safe riders. You make snowmobiling safe.

Snowmobiling is fun, but it's work, too. It challenges the body and mind, and that's part of the reason you're so relaxed at the end of a day of snowmobiling. While you are riding, the wind, sun, glare, cold, vibration, motion, and other factors work together to affect both driver and passenger.

Yes, there's plenty of challenge awaiting you as you drive your snowmobile into the winter wonderland. Alcohol magnifies and distorts those challenges

---

About This Chapter: "Snowmobiling Safety," © International Snowmobile Manufacturers Association (www.snowmobile.org). All rights reserved. Reprinted with permission. Available online at http://www.snowmobile.org/snowmobilesafety.asp, accessed April 29, 2008.

and can quickly turn an enjoyable outing into a situation that's hazardous for you and others.

Alcohol And Snowmobiling, Simply, Do Not Mix

Forget that myth that alcohol warms up a chilled person. It opens the blood vessels and removes the feeling of chill, but it does nothing to increase body heat. Instead, it can increase the risk of hypothermia, a dangerous lowering of the body's core temperature. With alcohol, you may only feel warmer, while your body chills dangerously.

Alcohol increases fatigue, fogs your ability to make good decisions, and slows your reaction time. It's part of a formula for disaster. And don't forget—most states and provinces have laws prohibiting the operation of a snowmobile while under the influence of alcohol.

As a safe rider, you:

- Know your abilities and don't go beyond them.
- Know your machine's capabilities and don't push beyond them.
- Know your riding area. Get a map. Talk to the local folks.
- Learn more—reading manuals and other materials from manufacturers, administrators, and snowmobile associations, or watch videos or computer programs from these sources. Snowmobile clubs, state, and provincial associations offer courses, information, and activities. Many members are certified driving or safety instructors.

Keep Your Machine In Top Shape

You have two good guides available for snowmobile maintenance: the owner's manual that came with it and your dealer. Consult both to make sure your machine is kept in top form for dependable, enjoyable fun.

Your local club or association may also conduct safety and maintenance programs.

Before each ride, follow the "pre-op" check outlined in your owner's manual.

Follow The Rules

Regulations on sled registration and use are different in various parts of the snow-belt. Check with natural resource and law enforcement agencies and snowmobile dealers or clubs in the area you are visiting to make sure your ride results in legal and hassle-free snowmobiling.

Remember, too, that some states and provinces have age restrictions for snowmobile operation, often requiring that children are supervised by adults.

Safe Crossing

Be careful when crossing roads of any kind. Come to a complete stop and make absolutely sure no traffic is approaching from any direction. Then cross at a right angle to traffic.

Dress Appropriately

Wear layers of clothing, so that you can add or remove a layer or two to match changing conditions. A windproof outer layer is especially important, as are warm gloves or mitts, boots, and a helmet.

Make sure your helmet is safety-certified, the right size, and in good condition. A visor is essential for clear vision and wind protection and the chin strap should be snug.

Wear glasses or goggles that offer protection from the sun.

Take A Friend

Don't snowmobile alone. Not only is snowmobiling more fun with family and friends, it's safer too.

File A Plan

Airplane pilots and boaters file flight and float plans, respectively, so that others know where to look if they're overdue.

"Snow plans" describing your machine and your planned route can be time- and life-savers. Leave only with your family or friends.

Like those who file travel plans, always let your family and friends know you're back or have arrived at your destination. No one likes needless searches.

Take Care Of The Trail

Safe riders snowmobile to enjoy the outdoors. They treat it with respect:

- They wait for enough snow cover to protect vegetation.
- They avoid running over trees and shrubs.
- They appreciate, but don't disturb, animals or other outdoor users.

Take The Honorable Trail

Beautiful trail systems and riding areas are available throughout North America. Stay safe and legal within the areas that you are permitted to ride or those for which you've obtained permission.

Stay Alert

Focusing on the tail light of the snowmobile ahead of you is the cause of many accidents. If your eyes are fixed on the tail light, you are not likely to notice the slight turn the machine ahead makes to avoid collision or the object that was almost hit.

> ♣ **It's A Fact!!**
> **A Good Turn**
>
> Other snowmobilers and car drivers need to know what you're up to. Remember the basic hand signals:
>
> - Left Turn: left arm extended straight out
> - Right Turn: left arm out, forearm raised, with elbow at 90-degree angle
> - Stop: left arm raised straight up
> - Slow: left arm out and angled toward ground

After snowmobiling for several hours, your reaction time slows. Be aware that even though you may not feel tired, the motion, wind and vibration of the machine may begin to dull your senses.

Beware Of Darkness

Low-light and darkness require special care. Slow down and watch for others. Overcast days require extra caution.

Snowmobile Safety

Don't over drive your headlights. Ask yourself, "Am I driving slow enough to see an object in time to avoid a collision?"

At night on lakes and large open fields, estimating distances and direction of travel may become difficult. It is important to keep some point of reference when riding at night.

Beware Of Water

The safest snowmobiling rule is never to cross lakes or rivers. Besides the danger of plunging through the ice, you have far less traction for starting, turning, and stopping on ice than on snow.

Collisions on lakes account for a significant number of accidents. Don't hold the attitude that lakes are flat, wide open areas, free of obstructions.

Remember, if you can ride and turn in any direction, without boundaries, so can other riders. The threat of a collision, then, can come from any direction.

However, if you do snowmobile on the ice, make absolutely sure the ice is safely frozen. Don't trust the judgment of other snowmobilers. You are responsible for your own safe snowmobiling. Drowning is a leading cause of snowmobile fatalities. Consider buying a buoyant snowmobile suit.

If you go through the ice, remember that your snowmobile suit (even a non-buoyant one) and helmet may keep you afloat for several minutes. Slide back onto the ice, using anything sharp to dig in for better pull. Kick your feet to propel you onto the ice, like a seal.

If the ice keeps breaking, continue moving toward shore or the direction from which you came. Don't remove your gloves or mitts.

Once on the ice, roll away from the hole. Don't stand until well away from the hole.

Mountain Measures

Even if we don't live near mountains, many of us want to visit the Cascades, Adirondacks, Rockies, or other mountains someday. Mountain snowmobiling is spectacular but can pose extra dangers, such as avalanches. Some avalanche areas may be posted and closed.

Be cautious of avalanche dangers throughout mountain country. Riding in these areas should only be done after receiving proper mountain riding training. Mountain snowmobilers should carry avalanche beacons, shovels, probe poles for locating people buried in snow, and a portable radio to summon help.

Join A Club

There are thousands of snowmobile clubs scattered throughout snow country, with associations or federations in every state and province.

Clubs sponsor outings and events year-around, monitor legislation, and speak up in public hearings. They also hold safety and maintenance workshops, build and care for trails, and publish newsletters.

Clubs can help law enforcement agencies and many raise funds for charity. For maximum snowmobiling fun—join a club. They are the backbone of the activity.

♣ It's A Fact!!
Avalanche Awareness

Following are some safe travel tips for riding in avalanche country:

- Learn to recognize and understand avalanche potential terrain. Suspect any slope that is steeper than 30 degrees.
- Observe the slope orientation with respect to the sun and the wind.
- Be cautious of cornices.
- Think about the consequences of an avalanche. Will you be carried over a cliff, pushed into trees or buried deep in a gully?
- Travel safely, ride with a partner, carry the appropriate rescue gear and make sure everyone in your group knows how to use it.
- For information on avalanche awareness please visit the website www.avalanche.org.

Chapter 49

Skating, Skateboarding, Skiing, And Snowboarding

Inline Skating

The latest innovation in roller skating is inline skating.

In 1980, inline skates were an ideal off-season training tool for hockey players. Inline skating spread from hockey players to skiers, who also used them for training, and then into the general population of fitness buffs and recreational sports consumers.

Swiftly gaining in popularity, rapid inline skating can burn as many calories per minute as cycling or running. Its low-impact, gliding strokes apply less injury-causing stress to the lower body joints than other sports such as aerobics or tennis. Ankles are well-protected because the boots are a heavy, thick plastic and rise above the ankle.

- About 20 million inline skaters hit the streets each year.
- According to the Consumer Product Safety Commission, as many as two-thirds of inline skaters do not wear safety gear.

About This Chapter: This chapter includes "Inline Skating," "Skateboarding Safety Tips," and "Ski and Snowboard Safety," © 2004 National Safety Council (www.nsc.org). Reprinted with permission.

- The Consumer Product Safety Commission estimates approximately 11,000 inline skaters suffer from head or face injuries annually.

- Inline skaters should always wear safety gear, including a helmet, knee and elbow pads, and wrist guards.

- Just as you would wear a helmet while bicycling, you should wear a helmet when inline skating.

- Helmets significantly reduce head and brain injury.

> ♣ **It's A Fact!!**
> Although many people know the sport as "rollerblading," the term Rollerblade® is a registered trademark of Rollerblade, Inc., and should not be used as a generic term for the sport. Accordingly, this document will refer to the equipment and sport by the generic terms "inline skates" and "inline skating," respectively.
>
> Source: "Inline Skating," © 2004 National Safety Council.

Since unintentional injuries can occur to even the most experienced inline skaters, the National Safety Council recommends these skating safety tips:

- Always wear protective equipment: elbow and knee pads, light gloves, helmets, and wrist guards.

- Before your first time out, take an inline skating course to learn the basics.

- Choose durable skates that match your needs, whether you exercise infrequently or race. Your plans will determine the type of skate you should buy.

- For proper ankle support, feel the plastic of the boot: if you can squeeze it, the material is not strong enough to give you reliable support.

- When buying skates, take socks to the store with you to ensure a proper fit, or buy the socks there.

- Begin skating with a five-minute, slow skate to warm up; you will be less likely to tear muscles.

- Start skating gradually on level ground. Practice moving forward, and ease into skating.

Skating, Skateboarding, Skiing, And Snowboarding

- While skating, keep knees slightly bent, which will lower your center of gravity and keep your body balanced on the balls of your feet.

- Practice stopping by bringing the foot with the heel stop forward until the heel stop is next to the toe of the other foot. Gently bend your front knee while lifting your toes up. This motion will bring you to a stop. This is known as the "heel stop." There are other stopping methods, such as T-stop and power stop, as well as several ways to slow down, for example, snowplowing and running on the grass.

Skaters should get current information on skating techniques and practice them for greatest enjoyment of the sport consistent with safety.

- Accept the fact that falls will happen and practice falling on a soft lawn or a gym mat if you are a novice skater.

- Be conscious of others: skaters, pedestrians, joggers, and bicyclists frequently use the same areas. To avoid collisions, use caution when skating around others.

- Skate on the right side of sidewalks, bike paths, and trails. Pass on the left as cars do, after yelling "passing on the left." Don't pass without warning. Also pass only when it is safe, and when you have enough room for both you and the person(s) you want to pass to be at the full extension position of your stroke.

- It is dangerous to skate in the street. In densely populated areas, be especially watchful for cars and other traffic when crossing roads and streets. Look left-right-left and cross when it is safe to do so. Remember that you must obey all traffic regulations.

- Watch for changes in skating trail conditions because of traffic, weather conditions, or hazards such as water, potholes or storm debris. When in doubt, slow down. Do not skate on wet or oily surfaces.

- Before using any trail, achieve a basic skating level, including the ability to turn, control speed, brake on downhills, and recognize and avoid skating obstacles.

- Check skates regularly to make sure they are in good condition. Replace worn wheels and the brake. Make sure the wheels are securely tightened and are not blocked by debris or grass.

Skateboarding Safety Tips

Skateboarding is a popular activity enjoyed by many young people. However, it's also an activity that causes many unintentional injuries.

According to the U.S. Consumer Product Safety Commission (CPSC), more than 15,600 persons need hospital emergency room treatment each year for injuries related to skateboarding. Fractures are a frequent type of injury. Deaths as a result of collisions with motor vehicles and from falls are also reported.

Irregular riding surfaces account for more than half of the skateboarding injuries caused by falls. Wrist injury is the number one injury, usually a sprain or a fracture. Skateboarders who have been skating for less than a week suffered one-third of the injuries. When experienced riders suffered injuries, it was usually from falls that were caused by rocks and other irregularities in the riding surface.

The National Safety Council offers these skateboarding tips:

The Skateboard/Protective Gear

- There are boards with varying characteristics for different types of riding; that is, slalom, freestyle, or speed. Some boards are rated as to the weight of the intended user.
- Protective equipment, such as closed, slip-resistant shoes, helmets, and specially designed padding, may not fully protect skateboarders from fractures, but wearing it can reduce the number and severity of cuts and scrapes.
- Padded jackets and shorts are available for skateboarders, as well as padding for hips, knees, and elbows. Wrist braces and special skateboarding gloves also can help absorb the impact of a fall.
- The protective equipment currently on the market is not subject to government performance standards and careful selection is necessary.

Skating, Skateboarding, Skiing, And Snowboarding

- In a helmet, look for proper fit and a chin strap; notice whether the helmet blocks vision and hearing. If padding is too tight, it could restrict circulation and reduce the ability to move freely. Loose-fitting padding, on the other hand, could slip off or slide out of position.

Tips For Using A Skateboard

- Give your board a safety check each time before you ride.
- Always wear safety gear.
- Never ride in the street.
- Obey the city laws. Observe traffic and areas where you can and cannot skate.
- Don't skate in crowds of non-skaters.
- Only one person per skateboard.
- Never hitch a ride from a car, bicycle, etc.
- Don't take chances; complicated tricks require careful practice and a specially designated area.
- Learn to fall—practice falling on a soft surface or grass.

> ### ✔ Quick Tip
> ### How To Fall
>
> Learning how to fall may help reduce the chances of a serious injury.
>
> - If you are losing your balance, crouch down on the skateboard so that you will not have as far to fall.
> - In a fall, the idea is to land on the fleshy parts of your body.
> - If you fall, try to roll rather than absorb the force with your arms.
> - Even though it may be difficult during a fall, try to relax your body, rather than go stiff.
>
> Source: "Skateboarding Safety Tips," © 2004 National Safety Council.

Ski And Snowboard Safely

Downhill skiing and snowboarding can be an exhilarating experience but, as with any sport, safety should come first. Excess speed and loss of control are the primary factors associated with snow skiing fatalities, according to a study reported in *The Physician and Sportsmedicine*, February 1989. The study also states that more than three-fourths of ski-related deaths occurred after collisions with stationary objects, such as trees and lift towers. Head injuries were cited most often as the cause of the fatalities. The National Safety Council strongly advises novice and experienced skiers and snowboarders to learn or reacquaint themselves with the proper skills and safety techniques.

Shaping-Up For The Season

Poor physical condition can be a contributing factor in skiing and snowboarding injuries. Being in good condition before attempting a strenuous sport will increase your enjoyment, reduce fatigue, and help avoid injury.

Getting in shape does not mean a "crash course" of exercising one week before a trip. A regular routine of exercise to strengthen muscles that will be used more than usual is recommended. You should start exercising well before the season starts. For exercises best suited to help you get in shape, consult a fitness expert or personal trainer.

Hitting The Slopes

A beginning skier or snowboarder should get proper instruction from a certified instructor before hitting the slopes. Among other basic skills, it is necessary to know how to fall down and get back up. At the start of the season, even an experienced skier or snowboarder should take a refresher course—just to be safe.

After you have mastered the basic skiing or snowboarding skills, the learning process is not over. Knowing snow conditions and the time of day you are planning to ski are just as important. Check with the local Ski Patrol for conditions and study a map of the area you will be skiing or snowboarding. Keep in mind that late in the day sunlight may obscure details of the terrain and make obstacles hard to see. One of the most important safety rules is to never ski or snowboard alone.

Selecting And Caring For Equipment

Always select and use quality equipment. Improperly fitted or mis-adjusted equipment can cause the best skier and snowboarder injury. When buying equipment ask for expert advice. A trained sales associate at a reputable ski and/or snowboard shop will be able to best assist you when purchasing equipment. If you own ski and/or snowboard equipment, have them checked for proper fit and adjustment periodically throughout the season.

> ♣ **It's A Fact!!**
>
> ## Rules Of The Slopes
>
> The following is a list of rules that all skiers and snowboarders should know and obey:
>
> - When skiing or snowboarding downhill, give moving skiers and snowboarders below the right of way. You should be able to see them: they might not see you.
> - Stop on the side of a run, well out of the way and in view of other skiers and snowboarders.
> - Look both ways and uphill before crossing a trail, merging or starting down the hill.
> - Use a safety device to prevent runaway equipment.
> - Never ski or snowboard alone.
> - Follow all posted signs and rules. Avoid closed trails and out-of-bound areas.
>
> Source: "Ski and Snowboard Safety," © 2004 National Safety Council.

Boots and bindings are the most important part of a ski or snowboard outfit. Boots should be snug and comfortable. Proper bindings are critical and should be checked by a professional regularly to make sure they are working properly. When purchasing skis or a snowboard, be sure to select the length and style right for your height and skill level.

Proper clothing is also an important part of your equipment. Choose comfortable, warm attire. Dress in layers. Bright colors are the best because they can be seen at a great distance. Outer wear should be made of a fabric which will reduce sliding after a fall and be water repellant.

Chapter 50

Thunderstorms: Take Cover

While thunder won't hurt you—lightning will. So it's important to pay attention when you hear thunder. Thunderstorms happen in every state and every thunderstorm has lightning. Lightning can strike people and buildings and is very dangerous.

Thunderstorms affect small areas when compared with hurricanes and winter storms. The typical thunderstorm is 15 miles in diameter and lasts an average of 30 minutes. Nearly 1,800 thunderstorms are happening at any moment around the world.

Despite their small size, all thunderstorms are dangerous. Every thunderstorm produces lightning, which kills more people each year than tornadoes. Heavy rain from thunderstorms can lead to flash flooding. Strong winds, hail, and tornadoes are also dangers associated with some thunderstorms. You can estimate how many miles away a storm is by counting the number of seconds between the flash of lightning and the clap of thunder. Divide the number of seconds by five to get the distance in miles. The lightning is seen before the thunder is heard because light travels faster than sound. (Of course, get safe shelter first, before you take the time to count the seconds.)

> About This Chapter: From "Thunderstorms," "Thunderstorms: If Someone Is Hit By Lightning," "Thunderstorms: Lightning Fact and Fiction," "Thunderstorms: Things to Know," and "Thunderstorms: What Is Lightning," undated publications of the Federal Emergency Management Agency (FEMA); available online at http://www.fema.gov/kids/thunder. Accessed February 5, 2008.

Thunderstorms are most likely to occur in the spring and summer months and during the afternoon and evening hours but they can occur year-round and at all hours of the day or night. Along the Gulf Coast and across the southeastern and western states, most thunderstorms occur during the afternoon. Thunderstorms often occur in the late afternoon and at night in the Plains states. Thunder and lightning can sometimes even come with snowstorm.

> ♣ **It's A Fact!!**
>
> Thunderstorms need three things:
> - Moisture—to form clouds and rain.
> - Unstable Air—relatively warm air that can rise rapidly.
> - Lift—fronts, sea breezes, and mountains are capable of lifting air to help form thunderstorms.

Things To Know

When a storm is coming, look for darkening skies, flashes of light, or increasing wind. Listen for the sound of thunder. If you can hear thunder, you are close enough to the storm to be struck by lightning. Go to safe shelter immediately. Find shelter in a building or car. Keep car windows closed and avoid convertibles.

Telephone lines and metal pipes can conduct electricity. Unplug appliances; avoid using the telephone or any electrical appliances. (Leaving electrical lights on, however, does not increase the chances of your home being struck by lightning.)

Don't take a bath or shower.

Turn off the air conditioner. Power surges from lightning can overload the compressor and damage the air conditioner.

Draw blinds and shades over windows. If windows break due to objects being blown by the wind of a storm, then the shades will prevent glass from shattering into your home.

If you are caught outside during a thunderstorm, you must act immediately:

Thunderstorms: Take Cover

- If you are in the woods, take shelter under the shorter trees.
- If you are boating or swimming, get to land and find shelter right away.
- If you can go to a low-lying, open place away from trees, poles, or metal objects. Make sure the place you pick is not subject to flooding.
- Become a very small target. Squat low to the ground. Place your hands on your knees with your head between them. Make yourself the smallest target possible.
- Do not lie flat on the ground—this will make you a larger target.

What Is Lightning?

The action of rising and descending air within a thunderstorm separates positive and negative charges. Water and ice particles also affect the distribution of electrical charge. Lightning results from the buildup and discharge of electrical energy between positively and negatively charged areas. Most lightning occurs within the cloud or between the cloud and ground.

The average flash of lightning could turn on a 100-watt light bulb for more than three months. The air near a lightning strike is hotter than the surface of the sun. The rapid heating and cooling of air near the lightning channel causes a shock wave that results in thunder.

Your chances of being struck by lightning are estimated to be one in 600,000 but those chances can be reduced by following safety rules. Most lightning deaths and injuries occur when people are caught outdoors, and most happen in the summer. Many fires in the western United States and Alaska are started by lightning. In the past 10 years, more than 15,000 fires have been started by lightning.

Lightning Fact And Fiction

Fiction: Lightning never strikes the same place twice.

Fact: Lightning has "favorite" sites that it may hit many times during one storm.

Fiction: If it is not raining, then there is no danger from lightning.

Fact: Lightning often strikes outside of heavy rain and may occur as far as 10 miles away from any rainfall.

Fiction: The rubber soles of shoes or rubber tires on a car will protect you from being struck by lightning.

Fact: Rubber-soled shoes and rubber tires provide no protection from lightning. However, the steel frame of a hard-topped vehicle provides increased protection if you are not touching metal. Although you may be injured if lightning strikes your car, you are much safer inside a vehicle than outside.

Fiction: People struck by lightning carry an electrical charge and should not be touched.

Fact: Lightning-strike victims carry no electrical charge and should be attended to immediately.

> ✔ **Quick Tip**
> **If Someone Is Hit By Lightning**
>
> People who have been struck by lightning are safe to handle—they don't carry an electrical charge.
>
> Call for help. Get someone to dial 911.
>
> Being struck by lightning can cause burns or nervous system damage, broken bones and loss of hearing and eyesight. It is a very serious emergency.
>
> If you know how, give first aid. If you know how and the person has stopped breathing, begin rescue breathing. If their heart has stopped beating, and you know how, give CPR.

Fiction: "Heat lightning" occurs after very hot summer days and poses no threat.

Fact: What is referred to as "heat lightning" is actually lightning from a thunderstorm too far away for thunder to be heard. However, the storm may be moving in your direction.

Part Six
Emergency And Disaster Preparedness

Chapter 51

Making A Disaster Plan

It's important to plan ahead so that during an emergency you know what to do and how to get in touch with other family members. Here's how to create a clear family emergency plan.

First, gather your family members (including your pets) together for a quick family meeting, maybe over a pizza or before watching your favorite movie.

Then, talk about the following questions and make a list of your family's solutions. Use the tips provided as a guide.

Before you know it you will have a plan in place that everyone in your family can follow. And if an unexpected event does happen you can stay calm; listen to the direction of adults around you, like your teachers or parents, and follow your plan.

The following topics can help you and your family discuss what you should do if there were an emergency and you were not together in the same place.

How would we get in touch with each other?

- Decide that each member will call or e-mail the same person. For example, each person will contact Uncle Bob first. If he's not home, each person will contact Aunt Suzie instead.

About This Chapter: The main text in this chapter includes excerpts from "Talk It Out" and "Family Supply List," undated documents produced by the U.S. Department of Homeland Security; available online at http://www.ready.gov/kids; accessed February 5, 2008.

> ♣ **It's A Fact!!**
>
> Every family needs to plan for what might happen. You should sit down with your family and talk about these kinds of things:
>
> - What types of disasters might happen
> - What you should do to prepare (like creating your family disaster kit)
> - What to do if you are asked to evacuate (which means to leave your home)
> - Where to meet away from your home in case of a fire (like a neighbor's house or the corner of the street)
> - Where to meet outside your neighborhood if you must evacuate. You should pick a friend or relative's house.
> - Where to call to "check in" if you become separated from your family during a disaster. You should memorize the phone number of a favorite aunt or family member who lives in another state. You would call there to report where you are so your family can find you.
>
> You can also talk with your whole neighborhood about disaster plans. Find out if someone in your neighborhood has a special skill—like being a doctor.
>
> Also, be sure your house has a smoke detector and remember to change the batteries twice a year. It's also a good idea to take a first aid class so you will be prepared to help others.
>
> Source: "Family Disaster Plan," Federal Emergency Management Agency (FEMA), undated.

- If cell phones are not working, you should try using a land-line phone at a neighbor's or friend's house, or a public telephone. Everyone should have coins or a prepaid phone card to make the call.
- It might be easier to reach a person who's out of town. You can contact him or her to let them know you're okay.

Where would we meet?

- Choose an easy-to-find location near your home, then practice getting there from different locations around your neighborhood.

Making A Disaster Plan

- Also, choose an easy-to-find location outside of your neighborhood in case you can't get home. With your parents, practice getting to that location from school, sports practice, or other places where you have after-school activities.

How would we remain in contact?

- You should keep a copy of your family's contact numbers and meeting place(s) taped to the inside of your binder or homework notebook, in your book bag, or your wallet. Your plan should include all the phone numbers you might need.

- Remember, you might have trouble getting through on the phone during an emergency. Just keep trying.

What would I do if I were at school?

- Make sure your parents talk to your teacher or school principal about the school's emergency plan.

- Depending on the unexpected event, your school may have a plan in place that will have you stay in your classroom or go somewhere else.

- The most important things you can do if an emergency happens while you are at school are to stay calm and listen to the direction of your teachers or principal.

What would we do about our pets?

- Visit the FEMA website (available online at http://www.fema.gov/kids/petkit.htm) to find out what pet-related items you will need to include in your supply kit.

- Make a plan for what you'll do with your pets if you can't take them with you. Remember, you may not be able to take them to a shelter.

Family Supply List

Emergency Supplies

Water, food, and clean air are important things to have if an emergency happens. Each family or individual's kit should be customized to meet specific

Fill out the following information for each family member and keep it up to date.

Name: _____ Name: _____

Date of Birth: _____ Date of Birth: _____

Important Medical Information: _____ Important Medical Information: _____

_____ _____

Name: _____ Name: _____

Date of Birth: _____ Date of Birth: _____

Important Medical Information: _____ Important Medical Information: _____

_____ _____

Where to go in an emergency. Write down where your family spends the most time: work, school and other places you frequent. Schools, daycare providers, workplaces, and apartment buildings should all have site-specific emergency plans

Home
Address: _____

Phone Number: _____

Evacuation Location: _____

Work
Address: _____

Phone Number: _____

Evacuation Location: _____

School
Address: _____

Phone Number: _____

Evacuation Location: _____

Work
Address: _____

Phone Number: _____

Evacuation Location: _____

Places you frequent
Address: _____

Phone Number: _____

Evacuation Location: _____

Places you frequent
Address: _____

Phone Number: _____

Evacuation Location: _____

Figure 51.1. Just In Case Family Plan, Part One.

Making A Disaster Plan

Important Information	Name	Telephone #
Doctor(s)		
Veterinarian/ Kennel:		
Other:		

Your family may not be together in an emergency, so plan how you will contact one another and review what you will do in different situations.

Out-of-State Contact Name: _____

Telephone Number: _____

Email: _____

Every family member should carry a copy of this important information:

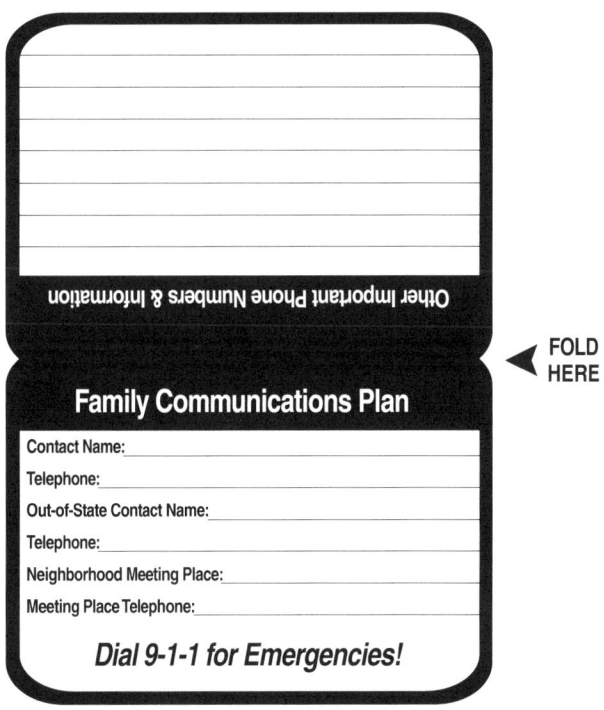

Figure 51.2. Just In Case Family Plan, Part Two.

> ✔ **Quick Tip**
> **Preparing Your Pets for Emergencies**
>
> If you are like millions of animal owners nationwide, your pet is an important member of your household. The likelihood that you and your animals will survive an emergency such as a fire or flood, tornado or terrorist attack depends largely on emergency planning done today. Some of the things you can do to prepare for the unexpected, such as assembling an animal emergency supply kit and developing a pet care buddy system, are the same for any emergency. Whether you decide to stay put in an emergency or evacuate to a safer location, you will need to make plans in advance for your pets. Keep in mind that what's best for you is typically what's best for your animals.
>
> If you must evacuate, take your pets with you if possible. However, if you are going to a public shelter, it is important to understand that animals may not be allowed inside. Plan in advance for shelter alternatives that will work for both you and your pets.
>
> Make a back-up emergency plan in case you can't care for your animals yourself. Develop a buddy system with neighbors, friends and relatives to make sure that someone is available to care for or evacuate your pets if you are unable to do so. Be prepared to improvise and use what you have on hand to make it on your own for at least three days, maybe longer.
>
> [Editor's Note: For more information about disaster preparedness for pets, see "Saving the Whole Family," produced by the American Veterinary Medical Association, available online at www.avma.org/disaster/saving_family.asp.]
>
> Source: "Preparing Your Pets for Emergencies Makes Sense. Get Ready Now." U.S. Department of Homeland Security, available online at www.ready.gov; accessed February 11, 2008.

needs, such as medications and infant formula. It should also be customized to include important family documents.

Recommended Supplies To Include In A Basic Kit

- Water, one gallon of water per person per day, for drinking and sanitation
- Food, at least a three-day supply of non-perishable food

Making A Disaster Plan

- Battery-powered radio and a National Oceanic and Atmospheric Administration (NOAA) Weather Radio with tone alert, and extra batteries for both
- Flashlight and extra batteries
- First aid kit
- Whistle to signal for help
- Infant formula and diapers, if you have an infant
- Moist wipes, garbage bags, and plastic ties for personal sanitation
- Dust mask or cotton t-shirt, to help filter the air
- Plastic sheeting and duct tape to shelter-in-place
- Wrench or pliers to turn off utilities
- Can opener for food (if kit contains canned food)

Clothing And Bedding

If you live in a cold weather climate, you must think about warmth. It is possible that the power will be out and you will not have heat. Rethink your clothing and bedding supplies to account for growing children and other family changes. One complete change of warm clothing and shoes per person, including the following:

- A jacket or coat
- Long pants
- A long sleeve shirt
- Sturdy shoes

> ♣ **It's A Fact!!**
> Every family should have a disaster supply kit in their home. The kit will help you and your family during a disaster. In a hurricane or earthquake, for example, you might be without electricity and the water supply may be polluted. In a heavy winter storm or flood, you may not be able to leave your house for a few days. In times like this, you will need to rely on yourself. Your disaster supply kit will make it easier. Remember, your family will probably never need to use your disaster supply kit, but it's always better to be prepared.
>
> Source: From "Disaster Supply Kit," Federal Emergency Management Agency (FEMA), undated.

- A hat and gloves
- A sleeping bag or warm blanket for each person

Below are some other items for your family to consider adding to its supply kit. Some of these items, especially those marked with an asterisk (*) can be dangerous, so please have an adult collect these supplies.

- Emergency reference material such as a first aid book or a print out of the information on www.ready.gov
- Rain gear
- Mess kits, paper cups, plates, and plastic utensils
- Cash or traveler's checks; change
- Paper towels
- Fire extinguisher
- Tent
- Compass
- Matches in a waterproof container*
- Signal flare*
- Paper, pencil
- Personal hygiene items including feminine supplies
- Disinfectant*
- Household chlorine bleach*—You can use bleach as a disinfectant (diluted nine parts water to one part bleach), or in an emergency you can also use it to treat water. Use 16 drops of regular household liquid bleach per gallon of water. Do not use scented, color safe, or bleaches with added cleaners.
- Medicine dropper
- Important family documents such as copies of insurance policies, identification, and bank account records in a waterproof, portable container.

Making A Disaster Plan

♣ **It's A Fact!!**
Get The News About Your Weather—
With A NOAA Weather Radio

Did you know there is a radio that broadcasts National Weather Service warnings and watches 24 hours a day—and warns you with an alarm of dangerous weather? It's true. It's called the NOAA Weather Radio network, and it's provided as a public service by the Department of Commerce's National Oceanic and Atmospheric Administration.

The NOAA Weather Radio network has more than 480 stations in the 50 states and in Puerto Rico, the U.S. Virgin Islands, and U.S. Pacific Territories.

How does the radio work? National Weather Service forecasters provide routine weather programming all the time to help you plan. The radios also send out a special alarm tone to alert you to a life-threatening situation. Why is that important? Sometimes, weather can turn deadly very fast. Tornadoes are the best example. Tornadoes may strike when people are sleeping or unaware of the forecast. Tornadoes can be deadly if people cannot seek an appropriate shelter—like a basement or an in-house safe room. With the NOAA Weather Radio, you will be alerted to dangerous weather with time to take shelter.

NOAA Weather Radios broadcast more than just warning about natural hazards. They also broadcast warnings and information and technological disasters, such as chemical releases or oil spills.

Every house should have a NOAA Weather Radio—just the way all houses should have a smoke detector. They can be purchased at stores that sell electronics. Most run on batteries or have battery back-up. Be sure to take it with you when you travel or are out boating or camping.

Be weather-safe. Have a NOAA Weather Radio.

Source: "NOAA Weather Radio," Federal Emergency Management Agency (FEMA), undated.

Chapter 52

Sheltering In Place: What It Means

What "Sheltering In Place" Means

Some kinds of chemical accidents or attacks may make going outdoors dangerous. Leaving the area might take too long or put you in harm's way. In such a case it may be safer for you to stay indoors than to go outside.

"Shelter in place" means to make a shelter out of the place you are in. It is a way for you to make the building as safe as possible to protect yourself until help arrives. You should not try to shelter in a vehicle unless you have no other choice. Vehicles are not airtight enough to give you adequate protection from chemicals.

Every emergency is different and during any emergency people may have to evacuate or to shelter in place depending on where they live.

How To Prepare To Shelter In Place

Choose a room in your house or apartment for the shelter. The best room to use for the shelter is a room with as few windows and doors as possible. A large room with a water supply is best—something like a master bedroom that is connected to a bathroom. For most chemical events, this room should be as high in the structure as possible to avoid vapors (gases) that sink. This

> About This Chapter: From "Chemical Agents: Facts About Sheltering in Place," Centers for Disease Control and Prevention, August 16, 2006.

guideline is different from the sheltering-in-place technique used in tornadoes and other severe weather and for nuclear or radiological events, when the shelter should be low in the home.

You might not be at home if the need to shelter in place ever arises, but if you are at home, the following items, many of which you may already have, would be good to have in your shelter room:

- First aid kit
- Flashlight, battery-powered radio, and extra batteries for both
- A working telephone
- Food and bottled water. Store one gallon of water per person in plastic bottles as well as ready-to-eat foods that will keep without refrigeration in the shelter-in-place room. If you do not have bottled water, or if you run out, you can drink water from a toilet tank (not from a toilet bowl). Do not drink water from the tap.
- Duct tape and scissors
- Towels and plastic sheeting. You may wish to cut your plastic sheeting to fit your windows and doors before any emergency occurs.

What To Do

Act quickly and follow the instructions of your local emergency coordinators such as law enforcement personnel, fire departments, or local elected leaders. Every situation can be different, so local emergency coordinators might have special instructions for you to follow. In general, do the following:

- Go inside as quickly as possible. Bring any outdoor pets indoors.
- If there is time, shut and lock all outside doors and windows. Locking them may pull the door or window tighter and make a better seal against the chemical. Turn off the air conditioner or heater. Turn off all fans, too. Close the fireplace damper and any other place that air can come in from outside.
- Go in the shelter-in-place room and shut the door.
- Turn on the radio. Keep a telephone close at hand, but don't use it unless there is a serious emergency.

> ♣ It's A Fact!!
> **How To Know If You Need To Shelter In Place**
> Most likely you will only need to shelter for a few hours.
> - If there is a "code red" or "severe" terror alert, you should pay attention to radio and television broadcasts to know right away whether a shelter-in-place alert is announced for your area.
> - You will hear from the local police, emergency coordinators, or government on the radio and on television emergency broadcast system if you need to shelter in place.

- Sink and toilet drain traps should have water in them (you can use the sink and toilet as you normally would). If it is necessary to drink water, drink stored water, not water from the tap.

- Tape plastic over any windows in the room. Use duct tape around the windows and doors and make an unbroken seal. Use the tape over any vents into the room and seal any electrical outlets or other openings.

- If you are away from your shelter-in-place location when a chemical event occurs, follow the instructions of emergency coordinators to find the nearest shelter. If your children are at school, they will be sheltered there. Unless you are instructed to do so, do not try to get to the school to bring your children home. Transporting them from the school will put them, and you, at increased risk.

- Listen to the radio for an announcement indicating that it is safe to leave the shelter.

- When you leave the shelter, follow instructions from local emergency coordinators to avoid any contaminants outside. After you come out of the shelter, emergency coordinators may have additional instructions on how to make the rest of the building safe again.

Chapter 53

Things To Know About Tornados, Hurricanes, And Floods

Tornados

Tornados are nature's most violent storms. Tornados must always be taken seriously. Tornados can be very dangerous—sometimes even deadly. They come from powerful thunderstorms and appear as rotating, funnel-shaped clouds. Tornado winds can reach 300 miles per hour. They cause damage when they touch down on the ground. They can damage an area one mile wide and 50 miles long. Every state is at some risk, but states in "Tornado Alley" have the highest risk. Tornados can form any time of the year, but the season runs from March to August. The ability to predict tornados is limited. Usually a community will have at least a few minutes warning. The most important thing to do is take shelter when a tornado is nearby.

What are tornados?

Tornados come from powerful thunderstorms and appear as rotating, funnel-shaped clouds with winds reaching up to 300 miles per hour. This is

> About This Chapter: Text in this chapter is from the following undated documents produced by the Federal Emergency Management Agency: "A Kid's Guide to Tornadoes and Preventing Disaster Damage," "Floods," "Fujita Pearson Tornado Scale," "Hurricane Classification," "Hurricanes," "Things to Know: Hurricanes," "Things to Know: Tornadoes," "Things to Know: Tsunamis," "Tornadoes," and "Tsunami." Available online at http://www.fema.gov/kids; accessed February 5, 2008.

about five times as fast as a car driving on a highway. Tornados cause damage when they touch down on the ground, and they can cause damage in areas one mile wide and 50 miles long. Severe weather can be very scary, and tornados are one of nature's most violent storms.

What should I do if a tornado is coming my way?

Tornados are hard to predict. Most of the time you will only have a few minutes warning. The most important thing to do is take cover when a tornado is nearby. It is also important to know the difference between a tornado watch and a tornado warning. A tornado watch is when tornados are possible in your area. No tornado has been spotted, but it could happen. A tornado warning is when a tornado has been seen, and you should take shelter immediately in a place without windows, such as your bathroom or your basement.

> ### What's It Mean?
>
> Tornado warning: A tornado has been sighted. Take shelter immediately.
>
> Tornado watch: Tornados are possible. Stay tuned to the radio or television news.
>
> Source: "Tornadoes," Federal Emergency Management Agency.

What should I know about tornados?

- Listen to a radio or watch television for weather updates. If a tornado is coming you must seek shelter. An underground shelter is best, such as a basement or storm shelter. If you don't have a basement, find an inside room or hallway or closet on the first floor away from windows.

- If you are at school during a tornado, listen and do what your teacher says.

- If you are outside and cannot get inside, lie flat in a ditch or ravine. Lie face down and cover your head with your hands.

- If you are in a car, take shelter in a nearby building.

- After a tornado, watch for broken glass and power lines that are downed. If you see people who are injured, don't move them unless they are in immediate danger. Call for help right away.

- Tornados can be very scary. If you are scared, be sure to talk to someone about it.

Hurricanes

Hurricanes are severe tropical storms that form in the southern Atlantic Ocean, Caribbean Sea, Gulf of Mexico, and in the eastern Pacific Ocean. Hurricanes gather heat and energy through contact with warm ocean waters. Evaporation from the seawater increases their power.

Hurricanes rotate in a counter-clockwise direction around an "eye." Hurricanes have winds at least 74 miles per hour. When they come onto land, the heavy rain, strong winds and heavy waves can damage buildings, trees, and cars. The heavy waves are called a storm surge. Storm surges are very dangerous and a major reason why you must stay away from the ocean during a hurricane warning or hurricane.

What should I know about hurricanes?

- Listen to a radio or television for weather updates and stay in touch with your neighbors about evacuation orders.
- Plan a place to meet your family in case you are separated during a disaster. Choose a friend or relative out of state for your family members to call to say they are OK.
- Assemble your disaster supplies kit. Store extra water now. Check to make sure you have enough food.
- Storm shutters are the best protection for windows. If your house does not have them, help an adult

♣ **It's A Fact!!**
Fujita Pearson Tornado Scale

F-0: 40–72 mph, chimney damage, tree branches broken

F-1: 73–112 mph, mobile homes pushed off foundation or overturned

F-2: 113–157 mph, considerable damage, mobile homes demolished, trees uprooted

F-3: 158–205 mph, roofs and walls torn down, trains overturned, cars thrown

F-4: 207–260 mph, well-constructed walls leveled

F-5: 261–318 mph, homes lifted off foundation and carried considerable distances, autos thrown as far as 100 meters

Source: From "Tornadoes," Federal Emergency Management Agency.

board up windows with 5/8" marine plywood. Tape does NOT prevent windows from breaking.

- Bring in outside furniture. An adult should remove roof antennas, if they can do so safely.

- Help an adult shut off your utilities—water, electricity, and gas.

- Make sure there is gas in the car and you are ready to evacuate immediately, if you are told to do so.

- If you don't need to evacuate, be sure to stay indoors during a hurricane. You could be hit by flying objects. Don't be fooled if there is a pause in the wind. It could be the eye of the storm, and the winds will come again.

- Avoid using the phone except for an emergency so the phone lines can stay open for others.

- If you do evacuate, do not go back home until local officials say it is safe.

- Hurricanes can be very scary. If you are scared, be sure to talk to someone about it.

How are hurricanes classified?

Hurricanes are classified into five categories, based on their wind speeds and potential to cause damage.

- Category One: Winds 74–95 miles per hour
- Category Two: Winds 96–110 miles per hour
- Category Three: Winds 111–130 miles per hour
- Category Four: Winds 131–155 miles per hour
- Category Five: Winds greater than 155 miles per hour

In the U.S., the official hurricane season is from June 1 to November 30, but hurricanes can happen any time of the year. Hurricanes are named by the National Weather Service. Some past hurricanes have been named: Opal, Andrew, Marilyn, Hugo, and Fran.

Tsunami

A tsunami is a series of huge waves that happen after an undersea disturbance, such as an earthquake or volcano eruption. (Tsunami is from the Japanese word for harbor wave.) The waves travel in all directions from the area of disturbance, much like the ripples that happen after throwing a rock. The waves may travel in the open sea as fast as 450 miles per hour. As the big waves approach shallow waters along the coast they grow to a great height and smash into the shore. They can be as high as 100 feet. They can cause a lot of destruction on the shore. They are sometimes mistakenly called "tidal waves," but tsunamis have nothing to do with the tides.

Hawaii is the state at greatest risk for a tsunami. They get about one a year, with a damaging tsunami happening about every seven years. Alaska is also at high risk. California, Oregon, and Washington experience a damaging tsunami about every 18 years.

> ### ❧ What's It Mean?
>
> Hurricane warning: A hurricane is expected within 24 hours. You may be told to evacuate. You and your family should begin making preparations to evacuate. If your area is having an evacuation, remember to take your disaster supply kit. Do not forget to make plans for your pets if you must evacuate.
>
> Hurricane watch: A hurricane is possible within 36 hours. Stay tuned to the radio and television for more information. The Hurricane Center is tracking the storm and trying to predict where it may come ashore.
>
> Source: "Hurricane," Federal Emergency Management Agency.

The Tsunami Warning Centers in Honolulu, Hawaii and Palmer, Alaska monitor disturbances that might trigger tsunami. When a tsunami is recorded, the center tracks it and issues a warning when needed.

What should I know about tsunamis?

If you feel an earthquake in the Pacific Coast area, turn on your battery-powered radio to learn if there is a tsunami warning. If you hear a tsunami warning, and they say to evacuate, do this immediately. You should have an evacuation plan.

A small tsunami at one beach can be a giant wave a few miles away. Do not let the small size of one wave make you forget how dangerous tsunami are. The next wave could be bigger. Get away from the shoreline right away. When you see a tsunami it is too late to escape. And stay away until you hear the "all clear" from officials. A tsunami is a series of waves, not a single wave, and the danger may not be over when you think it is.

Floods

Flooding happens during heavy rains, when rivers overflow, when ocean waves come onshore, when snow melts too fast or when dams or levees break. Flooding may be only a few inches of water or it may cover a house to the rooftop. Floods that happen very quickly are called flashfloods. Flooding is the most common of all natural hazards. It can happen in every U.S. state and territory.

> ♣ **It's A Fact!!**
>
> In 1964, an Alaskan earthquake generated a tsunami with waves between 10 and 20 feet high along parts of the California, Oregon, and Washington coasts.
>
> In 1946, a tsunami with waves of 20 to 32 feet crashed into Hilo, Hawaii, flooding the downtown area.
>
> Source: "Tsunami," Federal Emergency Management Agency.

◈ What's It Mean?

Flashflood warning: A flashflood is happening. Get to high ground right away. Tell an adult.

Flood warning: You may be asked to leave the area. A flood may be happening or will be very soon. Tell an adult if you hear a flood warning. If you have to leave the area, remember to bring your Disaster Supply Kit and make arrangements for your pets.

Flood watch or flashflood watch: Flooding may happen soon. Stay tuned to the radio or television news for more information. If you hear a flashflood warning, talk to an adult immediately.

Source: "Flood," Federal Emergency Management Agency.

Chapter 54

Be Prepared For Winter Storms

In many areas of the country, winters bring heavy snowfall and very cold temperatures. Heavy snow can block roads and cause power lines to fall down. The cold temperatures can be dangerous if you are not dressed correctly.

Winter Storms

- Be prepared for winter storms by having the following items:
    - a battery-powered radio with extra batteries
    - extra food that doesn't need cooking (like canned food)
    - rock salt to melt ice and sand to improve traction
    - flashlights and battery-powered lamps (if the electricity goes off)
    - wood for your fireplace (if you have one)
- If you go out in very cold weather, dress in several layers of clothing. Mittens are warmer than gloves, and you should wear a hat and cover your mouth with a scarf to protect your lungs from the cold air. Watch for frost bite. (Frostbite happens when your skin is exposed in very cold temperatures or you are not dressed warmly enough. You will have a loss of feeling in that part—usually a finger or toe or the tip of

---

About This Chapter: Text in this chapter is from the following undated documents produced by the Federal Emergency Management Agency: "Things to Know: Winter Storms," "Winter Storms," and "Winter Weather Makes Driving More Difficult." Available online at http://www.fema.gov/kids; accessed February 5, 2008.

your nose—and it may turn white or pale. Get help right away.)

- If you get trapped in your car during a blizzard, you should set your lights on flashing and hang a piece of cloth or distress flag from the radio antennae or window. Then get back in and stay in the car. Do not go out on foot unless you can see a building nearby. Run the engine and heater about 10 minutes out of each hour. When the engine is running, open a window slightly. This will protect you from carbon monoxide poisoning. You may need to clear snow away from the car's exhaust pipe.

- You can use road maps, seat covers, and floor mats for warmth. You can also huddle with the other passengers. Take turns sleeping so one person is always awake when rescuers come.

- If you are stranded in a remote area you may need to leave the car on foot after the blizzard passes.

Winter Weather Makes Driving More Difficult

Roads are slick and slippery, and falling snow or heavy rain can make it hard to see. And if your car breaks down in bad weather, the situation can get serious. Even though most kids aren't the ones doing the driving, it's still good for you to know how to be prepared for winter road conditions.

> ### 🕮 What's It Mean?
>
> Blizzard warning: Heavy snow and strong winds will produce a blinding snow, near zero visibility, deep drifts, and life-threatening wind chill.
>
> Freezing rain: Rain that freezes when it hits the ground, creating a coating of ice on roads and walkways.
>
> Frost/freeze warning: Below freezing temperatures are expected.
>
> Sleet: Rain that turns to ice pellets before reaching the ground. Sleet also causes roads to freeze and become slippery.
>
> Winter storm warning: Severe winter conditions have begun or will begin very soon.
>
> Winter storm watch: Severe weather such as heavy snow or ice is possible in the next day or two.
>
> Winter weather advisory: Cold, ice, and snow are expected.

For example, make sure you have the correct supplies in your family car. You should have in your trunk blankets, warm clothing, booster cables and tools, bottled water, canned fruits and nuts, a first aid kit, fire extinguisher, flashlight and batteries, traction mats or chains, a shovel, and ice scrapers. It's also a good idea to have a colorful scarf or piece of bright cloth to tie to your radio antennae to signal that you need help.

If you are caught in a storm or blizzard and your car becomes stuck, it is important to stay in the car and await rescue. Only leave the car and walk for help if you can see a definite safe-haven—like a house or a school—within a reasonable distance. When you are waiting in your car, turn on the engine for brief periods to provide heat, but always leave a down-wind window open slightly to avoid deadly carbon monoxide poisoning. Also, make sure the exhaust pipe is clear of snow. Leave the dome light on at night to signal rescuers, and exercise occasionally by clapping hands or moving around.

Natural disasters can play havoc with power lines and telephone poles. Be aware of your changed environment and stay away from downed power lines whether you are walking or driving.

Sometimes severe winter weather is followed by serious flooding. Never try to drive through water on a road. Water can be deeper than it seems and water levels can rise very quickly. A car can be lifted up by floodwaters and float out of control. Wade through floodwaters only if the water is not flowing rapidly and only in water no higher than the knees. If the car stalls in floodwater, get out quickly and move to higher ground (floodwaters may still be rising and the car could be swept away).

Share these driving tips with your family members who drive. They are very important. They could save a life.

Chapter 55

Earthquakes, Volcanoes, And Wildfires: What You Should Know

Earthquakes are the shaking, rolling, or sudden shock of the earth's surface. Earthquakes happen along "fault lines" in the earth's crust. Earthquakes can be felt over large areas although they usually last less than one minute. Earthquakes cannot be predicted—although scientists are working on it.

Most of the time, you will notice an earthquake by the gentle shaking of the ground. You may notice hanging plants swaying or objects wobbling on shelves. Sometimes you may hear a low rumbling noise or feel a sharp jolt. A survivor of the 1906 earthquake in San Francisco said the sensation was like riding a bicycle down a long flight of stairs.

The intensity of an earthquake can be measured. One measurement is called the Richter scale. Earthquakes below 4.0 on the Richter scale usually do not cause damage, and earthquakes below 2.0 usually can't be felt. Earthquakes over 5.0 on the scale can cause damage. A magnitude 6.0 earthquake is considered strong, and a magnitude 7.0 is a major earthquake.

About This Chapter: This chapter includes information from the following undated documents produced by the Federal Emergency Management Agency: "Earthquakes: Facts and Fiction," "Earthquakes: Home Hazards Hunt," "Things to Know: Earthquakes," "Things to Know: Volcanoes," ""Volcanoes," and "Wildfires." Available online at http://www.fema.gov/kids; accessed February 5, 2008.

Earthquakes are sometimes called temblors, quakes, shakers, or seismic activity. The most important thing to remember during an earthquake is to drop, cover, and hold on. So remember to drop to the floor and get under something for cover and hold on during the shaking.

Things To Know About Earthquakes

- If you are indoors during an earthquake, keep calm and take cover under a heavy table or desk. Stay away from glass, windows, or anything that could fall, like a bookcase.

- If you are outdoors, move away from buildings, street lights, and utility wires.

- If you are in a crowded public place, do NOT rush for the doors. Everyone will be doing that. Instead, take cover under something heavy and stay away from things that could fall on you. Stay calm. Do not get in an elevator during an earthquake.

- After an earthquake, be prepared for after shocks. After shocks are follow-up earthquakes that are usually smaller than the first one. They are dangerous because they can cause things that are weakened in the first earthquake to fall down.

- Make sure you are wearing shoes after an earthquake. There may be broken glass on the ground and inside your home.

Earthquakes: Home Hazards Hunt

- China cabinet; tall knickknack shelves; bookshelves (should be attached to wall studs)

- Heavy hanging plant over a place where people sit (should be light, unbreakable pot and make sure all plants hang from ceiling studs)

- A mirror on the wall (make sure it is well fastened to the wall)

- Heavy objects on wall shelves (should be moved to bottom shelves or secured)

- Unsecured TV on a rolling cart (make sure cart wheels are blocked so TV can't roll)

- Bed by a big window (bed should be moved away)
- Heavy picture above a bed (bed or picture should be moved)
- A hanging light above a bed (light should be secured with extra wire or chain, or the bed should be moved)
- Cabinet doors not fastened to stay closed (install latches)
- Unattached water heater (attach water heater to the wall studs)
- Gas stove with rigid feed line (replace gas line with flexible connectors)
- Heavy wall clock (attach to wall studs)
- Chimney (brace outside chimney to the house)
- House not bolted to the foundation (foundation should be bolted)

> ♣ **It's A Fact!!**
> **Earthquakes: Facts And Fiction**
>
> **Fiction:** Earthquakes usually happen in the morning.
>
> **Fact:** Earthquakes happen in both the day and the night. There is no pattern.
>
> **Fiction:** There is such a thing as "earthquake weath-er."
>
> **Fact:** There is no connection between earthquakes and weather. Remember, earthquakes happen deep in the earth, far away from the weather.
>
> **Fiction:** We can prevent earthquakes from happening.
>
> **Fact:** No. You can protect yourself by doing things to secure buildings, like your home, but earthquakes can't be prevented—or predicted.
>
> Source: "Earthquakes," Federal Emergency Management Agency.

Volcanoes

A volcano is a mountain that opens downward to a pool of molten rock below the surface of the earth. When pressure builds up, eruptions occur. Gases and rock shoot up through the opening and spill over or fill the air with lava fragments. Eruptions can cause lateral blasts, lava flows, hot ash flows, mudslides, avalanches, falling ash, and floods. Volcano eruptions have been known to knock down entire forests. An erupting volcano can trigger tsunamis, flashfloods, earthquakes, mudflows, and rockfalls.

♣ **It's A Fact!!**

Why talk about landslides?

Landslides are a serious geologic hazard common to almost every state in the United States. It is estimated that nationally they cause up to $2 billion in damages and from 25 to 50 deaths annually. Globally, landslides cause billions of dollars in damage and thousands of deaths and injuries each year. Individuals can take steps to reduce their personal risk. Know about the hazard potential where you live, take steps to reduce your risk, and practice preparedness plans.

What are landslides and debris flows, and what causes them?

Some landslides move slowly and cause damage gradually, whereas others move so rapidly that they can destroy property and take lives suddenly and unexpectedly. Gravity is the force driving landslide movement. Factors that allow the force of gravity to overcome the resistance of earth material to landslide movement include: saturation by water, steepening of slopes by erosion or construction, alternate freezing or thawing, earthquake shaking, and volcanic eruptions.

Landslides are typically associated with periods of heavy rainfall or rapid snow melt and tend to worsen the effects of flooding that often accompanies these events. In areas burned by forest and brush fires, a lower threshold of precipitation may initiate landslides.

Debris flows, sometimes referred to as mudslides, mudflows, lahars, or debris avalanches, are common types of fast-moving landslides. These flows generally occur during periods of intense rainfall or rapid snow melt. They usually start on steep hillsides as shallow landslides that liquefy and accelerate to speeds that are typi-

---

Active volcanoes in the U.S. are found mainly in Hawaii, Alaska, California, Oregon, and Washington. The greatest chance of eruptions near areas where many people live is in Hawaii and Alaska. The danger area around a volcano covers about a 20-mile radius. In May 18, 1980, Mount St. Helens erupted in Washington state. It killed 58 people and caused more than $1 billion in property damage.

Fresh volcanic ash, made of pulverized rock, can be harsh, acidic, gritty, glassy, and smelly. The ash can cause damage to the lungs of older people, babies, and people with respiratory problems.

Earthquakes, Volcanoes, And Wildfires

cally about 10 miles per hour, but can exceed 35 miles per hour. The consistency of debris flows ranges from watery mud to thick, rocky mud that can carry large items such as boulders, trees, and cars. Debris flows from many different sources can combine in channels, and their destructive power may be greatly increased. They continue flowing down hills and through channels, growing in volume with the addition of water, sand, mud, boulders, trees, and other materials. When the flows reach flatter ground, the debris spreads over a broad area, sometimes accumulating in thick deposits that can wreak havoc in developed areas.

Among the most destructive types of debris flows are those that accompany volcanic eruptions. A spectacular example in the United States was a massive debris flow resulting from the 1980 eruptions of Mount St. Helens, Washington. Areas near the bases of many volcanoes in the Cascade Mountain Range of California, Oregon, and Washington are at risk from the same types of flows during future volcanic eruptions.

Wildfires can also lead to destructive debris-flow activity. In July 1994, a severe wildfire swept Storm King Mountain, west of Glenwood Springs, Colorado, denuding the slopes of vegetation. Heavy rains on the mountain in September resulted in numerous debris flows, one of which blocked Interstate 70 and threatened to dam the Colorado River.

Learn whether landslides or debris flows have occurred in your area by contacting local officials, state geological surveys or departments of natural resources, and university departments of geology.

Source: This excerpt from "Landslide and Debris Flow (Mudslide)," is reprinted courtesy of the American National Red Cross, © 2008. All rights reserved.

Things To Know About Volcanoes

Do not visit the volcano site. You could be killed by a sudden explosion. Public officials may tell you where it is safe to view.

If there is ash in the air, avoid being downwind from the volcano. A building offers good shelter from volcanic ash, but not from lava flows or rocks. If ash is falling, stay indoors unless there is a danger of the roof collapsing. Close doors, windows, and all ventilation in the house. Cover your nose and mouth to avoid breathing ash.

Be aware of flying rocks and mudflows. Mudflows can move faster than you can walk or run.

If you live near a volcano, you should have an evacuation plan. Know what route you will take if you must evacuate and have a back-up route, too. Also, if you live near a volcano it is good to have a pair of goggles and a throw-away breathing mask for each member of your household.

After an eruption, if you have ash on your roof, clear it away as soon as you can. The ash is heavy and could cause the roof to collapse.

Wildfires

It is very important to prepare for both building fires and wild fires. Fires in buildings are very dangerous. Every year, about 5,000 people in this country are killed by building fires.

One of the most important things to remember is that your house should have a working smoke detector. Look around your house to see if you have a smoke detector on every floor in the house. Get help from a parent or adult to check if your smoke detectors are working. Check also to see if your family has a working fire extinguisher.

Your family should have a fire plan of how to escape from your house if it is on fire. If you are caught in a fire remember, stay low to the ground where the smoke is not so heavy. Never hide during a fire. Always get out. And once you are out, stay out. Do not go back for a toy. Tell an adult if there is a person left behind in the burning house.

Wildfires are a danger for people who live in forest, prairies, or wooded areas. These fires are sometimes started by lightning or by accident. They can move very fast and burn many acres. Remember, if there is a wildfire near you and your family is told to evacuate—go right away. And remember to bring your pets with you.

Chapter 56

Chemical Emergencies

Chemicals Are An Important Part Of Life

Chemicals are a natural and important part of our environment. Even though we often don't think about it, we use chemicals every day. Chemicals help keep our food fresh and our bodies clean. They help our plants grow and fuel our cars. And chemicals make it possible for us to live longer, healthier lives.

Under certain conditions, chemicals can be poisonous or have a harmful effect on your health. Some chemicals which are safe, and even helpful in small amounts, can be harmful in larger quantities or under certain conditions.

Chemical accidents do happen—at home and in the community, and the American Red Cross wants you to be prepared.

How You May Be Exposed To A Chemical

You may be exposed to a chemical in three ways:

- Breathing the chemical
- Swallowing contaminated food, water, or medication

About This Chapter: "Chemical Emergencies," is reprinted courtesy of the American Red Cross, © 2008. All rights reserved. Although the text in this chapter is addressed to parents, teens can still benefit from the suggestions and learn about topics they may wish to discuss with their parents.

- Touching the chemical, or coming into contact with clothing or things that have touched the chemical

Remember, you may be exposed to chemicals even though you may not be able to see or smell anything unusual.

Children And Poisoning

The most common home chemical emergencies involve small children eating medicines. Experts in the field of chemical manufacturing suggest taking hazardous materials out of sight could eliminate up to 75 percent of all poisoning of small children.

> ♣ **It's A Fact!!**
> **Chemical Accidents Can Be Prevented**
> Many people think of chemicals as only those substances used in manufacturing processes. But chemicals are found everywhere—in our kitchens, medicine cabinets, basements, and garages. In fact, most chemical accidents occur in our own homes. And they can be prevented.

Keep all medicines, cosmetics, cleaning products, and other household chemicals out of sight and out of reach of children. If your child should eat or drink a non-food substance, find any containers immediately and take them to the phone. Call the Poison Control Center (800-222-1222) or Emergency Medical Services (EMS), or 9-1-1, if you have it in your area, or call the operator giving this information.

Follow their instructions carefully. Often the first aid advice found on containers may not be appropriate. So, do not give anything by mouth until you have been advised by medical professionals.

Home Product Precautions

Other home accidents can result from trying to improve the way a product works by adding one substance to another, not following directions for use of a product, or by improper storage or disposal of a chemical.

The first precaution you can take is to avoid mixing common household chemical products. Some combinations of these products, such as ammonia and bleach, can create toxic gases.

Chemical Emergencies

A second important precaution is to always read the directions before using a new product. Some products should not be used in a small confined space to avoid inhaling dangerous vapors. Other products should not be used without gloves and eye protection to help prevent the chemical from touching your body. Read and follow the directions.

Another effective way to protect yourself and your family is to store chemical products properly. Non-food products should be stored tightly closed in their original containers so you can always identify the contents of each container and how to properly use the product.

Never smoke while using household chemicals. Don't use hair spray, cleaning solutions, paint products, or pesticides near the open flame of an appliance, pilot light, lighted candle, fireplace, wood burning stove, etc. Although you may not be able to see or smell them, vapor particles in the air could catch fire or explode.

If you should spill a chemical, clean it up immediately with some rags, being careful to protect your eyes and skin. Allow the fumes in the rags to evaporate outdoors in a safe place, then dispose of them by wrapping them in a newspaper and then placing them in a sealed plastic bag. Dispose of these materials with your trash. If you don't already have one, buy a fire extinguisher that is labeled for A, B, and C class fires and keep it handy.

Buy only as much of a chemical as you think you will use. If you have product left over, try to give it to someone who will use it. Take care to dispose of it properly. Improper disposal can result in harm to yourself or members of your family, accidentally contaminate our local water supply, or harm other people.

It is also important to dispose of products properly to preserve our environment and protect wildlife. Plus, some products can be recycled and further protect our environment.

Many household chemicals can be taken to your local household hazardous waste collection facility. Many facilities accept pesticides, fertilizers, household cleaners, oil-based paints, drain and pool cleaners, antifreeze, and brake fluid. If you have questions about how to dispose of a chemical, call the facility or the environmental or recycling agency to learn the proper method of disposal.

Disaster Plan

Making a disaster plan will help each family member to stay calm in an emergency. But most important, planning ahead can save the lives of the people you love. The plan should include what task each family member is responsible for during an emergency, where supplies are kept, how family members will let one another know where they are going if they are evacuated, and where everyone will meet when the disaster is over.

Family Disaster Supplies Kit

A family disaster plan should include a family disaster supplies kit. Let each member of the family help put it together. The kit should include:

- a first aid kit;
- a battery-operated radio, flashlight, and extra batteries;
- bath size towels;
- plastic garbage bags;
- wide tape;
- a county map;
- bottled water (at least three gallons of water per person);
- non-perishable snack food; and
- a list of family medications, eyeglasses, and hearing aids.

Ask one person to be responsible for replacing water every three months and food every six months. Batteries should also be replaced on a regular basis.

Tape the call letters and frequency numbers of your emergency alert radio stations (EAS) on the radio and make sure everyone knows how to work the radio and put in fresh batteries. Also tape the channel number of the television emergency broadcast stations on your TV.

Every member of the family should know where the family disaster supplies kit is located—it should be stored within easy reach.

Chemical Emergencies

If you are a parent, don't assume that you will always be with your children in an emergency. Make sure they know how to protect themselves if you are not available to help.

At the beginning of the school year, take time to study the school or day care center emergency protective action plan, and discuss it with your children and their babysitters.

Major Chemical Emergencies

A major chemical emergency is an accident that releases a hazardous amount of a chemical into the environment. Accidents can happen underground, on railroad tracks or highways, and at manufacturing plants. These accidents sometimes result in a fire or explosion, but many times you cannot see or smell anything unusual.

How You May Be Notified Of A Major Chemical Emergency

In the event of a major chemical emergency, you will be notified by the authorities. To get your attention, a siren could sound, you may be called by telephone, or emergency personnel may drive by and give instructions over a loudspeaker. Officials could even come to your door.

Listen carefully to radio or television emergency alert stations (EAS), and strictly follow instructions. Your life could depend on it. You will be told:

- the type of health hazard;
- the area affected;
- how to protect yourself;
- evacuation routes (if necessary);
- shelter locations;
- type and location of medical facilities; and
- the phone numbers to call if you need extra help.

Do not call the telephone company, and do not call EMS, 9-1-1, or the operator for information. Dial these numbers only for a possible life-threatening emergency.

> ♣ **It's A Fact!!**
>
> **Shelter In Place**
>
> One of the basic instructions you may be given in a chemical emergency is to "shelter in place". This is a precaution aimed to keep you and your family safe while remaining in your home. If you are told to shelter in place, take your children and pets indoors immediately.
>
> While gathering your family, you can provide a minimal amount of protection to your breathing by covering your mouth and nose with a damp cloth.
>
> - Close all windows in your home.
> - Turn off all fans, heating, and air conditioning systems.
> - Close the fireplace damper.
> - Go to an above-ground room (not the basement) with the fewest windows and doors.
> - Take your family disaster supplies kit with you.
> - Wet some towels and jam them in the crack under the doors.
> - Tape around doors, windows, exhaust fans, or vents. Use the plastic garbage bags to cover windows, outlets, and heat registers.
> - If you are told there is danger of explosion, close the window shades, blinds, or curtains. To avoid injury, stay away from the windows.
> - Stay in the room and listen to your radio until you are told all is safe or you are told to evacuate.

Evacuation

Authorities may decide to evacuate an area for your protection. Again, it is important to stay calm, listen carefully and follow all instructions.

If you are told to evacuate, listen to your radio to make sure the evacuation order applies to you and to understand if you are to evacuate immediately or if you have time to pack some essentials. Do not use your telephone.

If you are told to evacuate immediately:

- take your disaster supplies kit and medications;
- close and lock your windows;

Chemical Emergencies 375

- shut off all vents;
- lock the door; and
- move quickly and calmly.

If the authorities tell you to evacuate because of a possible chemical emergency, take your family disaster supplies kit: a change of clothing for each member of the family; medication, eyeglasses, hearing aids or dentures, or things like canes and walkers; personal items such as toothbrushes, deodorant, etc.; items for your baby such as diapers, formula, or baby food; and books, puzzles, or cards and games for entertainment.

- Do not assume that a shelter will have everything you need. In most cases, the shelters will provide only emergency items such as meals, cots, and blankets.
- You don't need to turn off your refrigerator or freezer, but you should turn off all other appliances and lights before locking your home as you leave.
- Check on neighbors to make sure they have been notified, and offer help to those with disabilities or other special needs. If you need a ride, ask a neighbor. If no neighbor is available to help you, listen to the emergency broadcast station for further instructions.
- Take only one car to the evacuation site.
- Close your car windows and air vents and turn off the heater or air conditioner.
- Don't take shortcuts because a shortcut may put you in the path of danger. For your safety, follow the exact route you are told to take.

Chemical Poisoning

There are several symptoms of chemical poisoning whether by swallowing, touching, or breathing:

- Difficulty breathing
- Changes in skin color
- Headache or blurred vision

- Dizziness
- Irritated eyes, skin, throat
- Unusual behavior
- Clumsiness or lack of coordination
- Stomach cramps or diarrhea

If you think you have been exposed to a toxic chemical, call the Poison Control Center (800-222-1222), EMS or 9-1-1, or the operator, whichever applies to your area.

If you see or smell something that you think may be dangerous, or find someone who has been overcome with toxic vapors, your first job is to make sure that you don't become a victim. If you remain in a dangerous area and become injured or unconscious, you cannot help yourself or any victims.

Because chemical poisoning can be a life-threatening emergency:

- send someone to call EMS, immediately.
- tell the operator the location of the emergency and the phone number from where you are calling.
- describe what has happened, how many people are involved, and what is being done to help.
- stay on the phone until the operator tells you to hang up.

If you are trained in CPR or first aid, and feel confident that you are not in danger, check the person for life-threatening injuries. Administer appropriate treatment, and then deal with the chemical injuries.

If you have not recently taken a course in CPR or first aid, contact your local Red Cross for course information and schedules.

> ♣ **It's A Fact!!**
> **Emergency Procedures For School Children**
>
> In an emergency, your children may be sheltered in place or evacuated from school. If protective actions are being taken at your children's school, do not go to the school. School personnel are trained to handle emergencies.
>
> Do not call your child's school. You could tie up a phone line that is needed for emergency communications.
>
> For further information, listen to local emergency radio and TV stations to learn when and where you can pick up your children.

Chemical Emergencies

First Aid Treatment For Chemical Burns

A chemical burn can be minor or life threatening, but proper treatment can reduce the chance of infection and the damage caused by contact with the chemical.

Remove any affected clothing or jewelry from the injury. Use lots of cool running water to flush the chemical from the skin until emergency help arrives. The running water will dilute the chemical fast enough to prevent the injury from getting worse.

Use the same treatment for eye burns and remove any contact lenses. Be careful to flush the eye from the nose outward.

If no large amount of clean water is available, gently brush the chemical off the skin and away from the victim and you.

If the chemical is on the face, neck, or shoulders, ask the victim to close his or her eyes before brushing off the chemical.

Cover the wound very loosely with a dry, sterile, or clean cloth so that the cloth will not stick to the wound. Do not put any medication on the wound. Seek medical attention immediately.

If you believe you have been contaminated with a chemical, call the Poison Control Center (800-222-1222), EMS, 9-1-1, or the operator immediately. If medical help is not immediately available, remove your clothing starting from the top and working your way down to your socks. Take care not to touch your contaminated clothing to your bare skin. Place your clothing in a plastic bag so it cannot contaminate other people or things. Take a thorough shower to wash any chemical away. Re-dress in clean clothing and go for medical help at your first opportunity.

Who Helps In A Chemical Emergency

There are many organizations that help the community in an emergency, such as police, fire, and sheriff departments, the American Red Cross, and government agencies. All these groups coordinate their activities through the local office of emergency management. In many areas there are local

Hazardous Materials, or Haz-Mat, Teams, who are trained to respond to chemical accidents. In the event of a chemical emergency, it is very important that you follow the instructions of these highly trained professionals. They know best how to protect you and your family.

The American Red Cross is an organization managed by volunteers from your community. Although it receives no money from the government, it is chartered by the U.S. Congress to provide disaster relief. All help given to people during a chemical, house fire, storm, or other emergency is free of charge and supported through charitable contributions and the United Way.

Emergency help may include shelter, meals, replacement of essential medication, and personal hygiene supplies. The Red Cross may also help reunite families by staying in touch with all evacuation sites.

The strength of the Red Cross is its core of volunteers who work in all levels of the organization. If you would like more information about becoming a Red Cross volunteer, either in Disaster Services, Health and Safety, Blood Services, or community programs, call your local Red Cross chapter.

Important Telephone Numbers Emergency Medical Service: 9-1-1

If an accident involving hazardous materials occurs, you will be notified by the authorities as to what steps to take. You may hear a siren, be called by telephone, or emergency personnel may drive by and give instructions over a loudspeaker. Officials could even come to your door. If you hear a warning signal, you should go indoors and listen to a local Emergency Alert System (EAS) station for emergency instructions from county or state officials. Ask your local office of emergency management or Red Cross chapter which stations carry official messages in your community.

Your local Red Cross chapter can provide additional materials in English and Spanish:

- "Your Family Disaster Plan" (ARC 4466) (available online at http://www.redcross.org/services/disaster/0,1082,0_601_,00.html)
- "Your Family Disaster Supplies Kit" (ARC 4463) (available online at http://www.redcross.org/services/disaster/0,1082,0_3_,00.html)

Chemical Emergencies

- "Home Chemical Safety and Emergency Procedures" Video (ARC 5045V)

> ☞ **Remember!!**
>
> ## Important Points To Remember
>
> - Chemicals are everywhere. They are an important part of life.
> - The most common chemical accidents occur in our own homes and can be prevented.
> - The best ways to avoid chemical accidents are to read and follow the directions for use, storage, and disposal of the product.
> - Don't mix products, especially household cleaning products.
> - Develop a family disaster plan and pack a family disaster supplies kit.
> - In the event of an emergency, follow the instructions of the authorities carefully. Listen to your emergency broadcast stations on radio and TV.
> - Use your phone only in life-threatening emergencies, and then call the Poison Control Center (800-222-1222), EMS, 9-1-1, or the operator immediately.
> - If you are told to "shelter in place," go inside, close all windows and vents and turn off all fans, heating or cooling systems. Take family members and pets to a safe room, seal windows and doors, and listen to emergency broadcast stations for instructions.
> - If you are told to evacuate immediately, take your family disaster supplies kit. Pack only the bare essentials, such as medications, and leave your home quickly. Follow the traffic route authorities recommend. Don't take short cuts on the way to the shelter.
> - If you find someone who appears to have been injured from chemical exposure, make sure you are not in danger before administering first aid.
> - And lastly, remember, the best way to protect yourself and your family is to be prepared.

Chapter 57

National Security Emergencies

Homeland Security Advisory System

Homeland Security Advisory System was designed after 9/11 to provide warnings to the American people about the threat level for a terrorist attack. There are five "threat conditions," and each has a specific color. Your federal government and emergency managers have specific actions they take depending on the threat level. The greater the risk of a terrorist attack, the higher the threat level.

Who decides what the threat level is? The nation's Attorney General and the Secretary for Homeland Security make that decision. These are the levels:

- **Low Condition (Green):** There is a low risk of terrorist attacks.

- **Guarded Condition (Blue):** There is a general risk of terrorist attacks.

- **Elevated Condition (Yellow):** There is a significant risk of terrorist attacks. The public should be alert to suspicious activity.

About This Chapter: This chapter includes excerpts from the following undated documents produced by the Federal Emergency Management Agency: "Homeland Security Advisory System," "National Security Emergencies: Things to Know," "What to Do If There Is a Chemical and Biological Attack," "What to Do If There Is a Nuclear or Radiological Attack," and "What to Do If There Is an Explosion." Available online at http://www.fema.gov/kids/nse; accessed February 5, 2008.

- **High Condition (Orange):** There is a high risk of terrorist attacks. Officials will take additional precautions at public events and restrict access to some specific sites within a city or area.

- **Severe Condition (Red):** There is a severe risk of terrorist attacks and is the highest level. Officials may close public and government buildings, activate special teams, and limit transportation systems. People should avoid public gathering places and stay tuned to the media.

Things To Know

You don't have to be afraid, but it's always a good idea to be aware of your surroundings. That means, notice if something around you doesn't seem quite right. Know where exits are in a building. Don't accept packages from strangers and don't touch any suspicious packages. If you are asked to evacuate a building, even in a drill, take it seriously. Get far away from windows or glass doors and get under another kind of shelter if possible. Follow the directions of the officials on the scene—and stay out of the way of the emergency officials who may be responding to the area.

What To Do If There Is An Explosion

If you are in a building that has an explosion—first, stay calm. You are in charge of yourself and you can get out. You should leave the building as quickly as possible. Do not stop to get books or toys or anything or to make a phone call. If things are falling around you, get under a sturdy table or desk until they stop falling. Then leave quickly, watching for weakened floors and stairs as you leave.

If there is a fire:

- Stay low to the floor and get out as quickly as possible.
- Cover your nose and mouth with a wet cloth.
- When approaching a closed door, use the back of your hand to feel parts of the door. If the door is not hot, open slowly and check to see if fire or smoke is blocking your escape route. If not, get out by crawling, if you need to. If your escape route is blocked, shut the door right away

National Security Emergencies

and find another way out, such as a window. If the door is hot, don't open it. Escape through a window. If you cannot escape, hang something to signal to firefighters that you need to be rescued.

- Since smoke and poisonous gases collects along the ceiling, stay low at all times.

What To Do If There Is A Chemical And Biological Attack

What are chemical weapons? They are poisonous vapors, aerosols, liquids, or solids that are toxic to people, animals, or plants. It's important to know that chemical agents are deadly but very difficult to deliver and produce. There has never been a chemical weapon attack in the U.S.

What are biological weapons? They are organisms or toxins that can kill or injure people, livestock and crops. The three basic groups of biological agents that might be used as weapons are bacteria, viruses and toxins. It's important to remember that most biological agents are difficult to grow and maintain.

If there is a chemical or biological weapon attack near you, authorities will tell you what to do.

Listening to the radio or television is a good way to know what authorities want people to do. Authorities may tell you to evacuate right away and to take shelter at a specific place, or they may tell you to stay exactly where you are and seal off the building or room. Staying in place is called "sheltering in place." So it's important to remember that you may not always evacuate in such an attack, as leaving may put you at greater risk.

♣ It's A Fact!!

If you are trapped under debris:

- Don't move round or kick up dust. Cover your mouth with a handkerchief or clothing.

- Tap over and over on a pipe or wall so that rescuers can hear where you are. Shout only as a last resort when you hear sounds of rescuers and think someone will hear you. Shouting might make you breath dangerous amounts of dust.

- Try to think of things that make you happy and stay calm. Rescuers are on the way.

What To Do If There Is A Nuclear Or Radiological Attack

Nuclear explosions can cause blinding light, intense heat, fires, and radiation fallout. You may have heard the term "dirty bomb," as a terrorist weapon. A "dirty bomb" is an explosive device that scatters radioactive material. You may have also heard the term "suitcase bomb," which is a very small nuclear device about the size of a suitcase. If the U.S. government knows of a threat of nuclear or radiological attack, officials will warn residents and may advise people to take cover or evacuate. Taking shelter during a nuclear attack is absolutely necessary—below ground is best. Stay there until officials say you can leave. Talk to your parents about the location of a possible shelter and have your parents talk to your school officials, too.

Chapter 58

Terrorism: Preparing For The Unexpected

Devastating acts, such as the terrorist attacks on the World Trade Center and the Pentagon, have left many concerned about the possibility of future incidents in the United States and their potential impact. They have raised uncertainty about what might happen next, increasing stress levels. Nevertheless, there are things you can do to prepare for the unexpected and reduce the stress that you may feel now and later should another emergency arise. Taking preparatory action can reassure you and your children that you can exert a measure of control even in the face of such events.

What You Can Do To Prepare

Finding out what can happen is the first step. Once you have determined the events possible and their potential in your community, it is important that you discuss them with your family or household. Develop a disaster plan together.

1. **Create an emergency communications plan:** Choose an out-of-town contact your family or household will call or e-mail to check on each other should a disaster occur. Your selected contact should live far enough away that they would be unlikely to be directly affected by the same event, and they should know they are the chosen contact. Make sure every household

---

About This Chapter: "Terrorism—Preparing for the Unexpected," is reprinted courtesy of the American National Red Cross, © 2008. All rights reserved. Although the text in this chapter is addressed to parents, teens can still benefit from the suggestions and learn about topics they may wish to discuss with their parents.

member has that contact's, and each other's, e-mail addresses and telephone numbers (home, work, pager, and cell). Leave these contact numbers at your children's schools, if you have children, and at your workplace. Your family should know that if telephones are not working, they need to be patient and try again later or try e-mail. Many people flood the telephone lines when emergencies happen but e-mail can sometimes get through when calls don't.

> ♣ **It's A Fact!!**
> Copies of essential documents—like powers of attorney, birth and marriage certificates, insurance policies, life insurance beneficiary designations and a copy of your will—should also be kept in a safe location outside your home. A safe deposit box or the home of a friend or family member who lives out of town is a good choice.

2. **Establish a meeting place:** Having a predetermined meeting place away from your home will save time and minimize confusion should your home be affected or the area evacuated. You may even want to make arrangements to stay with a family member or friend in case of an emergency. Be sure to include any pets in these plans, since pets are not permitted in shelters and some hotels will not accept them.

3. **Assemble a disaster supplies kit:** If you need to evacuate your home or are asked to "shelter in place," having some essential supplies on hand will make you and your family more comfortable. Prepare a disaster supplies kit in an easy-to-carry container such as a duffel bag or small plastic trash can. Include "special needs" items for any member of your household (infant formula or items for people with disabilities or older people), first aid supplies (including prescription medications), a change of clothing for each household member, a sleeping bag or bedroll for each, a battery powered radio or television and extra batteries, food, bottled water, and tools. It is also a good idea to include some cash and copies of important family documents (birth certificates, passports, and licenses) in your kit.

4. **Check on the school emergency plan of any school-age children you may have:** You need to know if they will they keep children at school until a parent or designated adult can pick them up or send them home on their own. Be sure that the school has updated information about how to reach

parents and responsible caregivers to arrange for pickup. And, ask what type of authorization the school may require to release a child to someone you designate, if you are not able to pick up your child. During times of emergency the school telephones may be overwhelmed with calls.

If Disaster Strikes

- Remain calm and be patient.
- Follow the advice of local emergency officials.
- Listen to your radio or television for news and instructions.
- If the disaster occurs near you, check for injuries. Give first aid and get help for seriously injured people.
- If the disaster occurs near your home while you are there, check for damage using a flashlight. Do not light matches or candles or turn on electrical switches. Check for fires, fire hazards, and other household hazards. Sniff for gas leaks, starting at the water heater. If you smell gas or suspect a leak, turn off the main gas valve, open windows, and get everyone outside quickly.
- Shut off any other damaged utilities.
- Confine or secure your pets.
- Call your family contact—do not use the telephone again unless it is a life-threatening emergency.
- Check on your neighbors, especially those who are elderly or disabled.

A Word On What Could Happen

As we learned from the events of September 11, 2001, the following things can happen after a terrorist attack:

- There can be significant numbers of casualties and/or damage to buildings and the infrastructure. So employers need up-to-date information about any medical needs you may have and on how to contact your designated beneficiaries.
- Heavy law enforcement involvement at local, state, and federal levels follows a terrorist attack due to the event's criminal nature.

- Health and mental health resources in the affected communities can be strained to their limits, maybe even overwhelmed.

- Extensive media coverage, strong public fear, and international implications and consequences can continue for a prolonged period.

- Workplaces and schools may be closed, and there may be restrictions on domestic and international travel.

- You and your family or household may have to evacuate an area, avoiding roads blocked for your safety.

- Clean-up may take many months.

Evacuation

If local authorities ask you to leave your home, they have a good reason to make this request, and you should heed the advice immediately. Listen to your radio or television and follow the instructions of local emergency officials and keep these simple tips in mind:

1. Wear long-sleeved shirts, long pants, and sturdy shoes so you can be protected as much as possible.

2. Take your disaster supplies kit.

3. Take your pets with you; do not leave them behind. Because pets are not permitted in public shelters, follow your plan to go to a relative's or friend's home, or find a "pet-friendly" hotel.

4. Lock your home.

5. Use travel routes specified by local authorities—don't use shortcuts because certain areas may be impassable or dangerous.

6. Stay away from downed power lines.

Listen To Local Authorities

Your local authorities will provide you with the most accurate information specific to an event in your area. Staying tuned to local radio and television, and following their instructions is your safest choice.

If you're sure you have time:

- Call your family contact to tell them where you are going and when you expect to arrive.
- Shut off water and electricity before leaving, if instructed to do so. Leave natural gas service on unless local officials advise you otherwise. You may need gas for heating and cooking, and only a professional can restore gas service in your home once it's been turned off. In a disaster situation it could take weeks for a professional to respond.

Additional Positive Steps You Can Take

Raw, unedited footage of terrorism events and people's reaction to those events can be very upsetting, especially to children. We do not recommend that children watch television news reports about such events, especially if the news reports show images over and over again about the same incident. Young children do not realize that it is repeated video footage and think the event is happening again and again. Adults may also need to give themselves a break from watching disturbing footage. However, listening to local radio and television reports will provide you with the most accurate information from responsible governmental authorities on what's happening and what actions you will need to take. So you may want to make some arrangements to take turns listening to the news with other adult members of your household.

> ♣ **It's A Fact!!**
> **Shelter-In-Place**
>
> If you are advised by local officials to "shelter in place," what they mean is for you to remain inside your home or office and protect yourself there. Close and lock all windows and exterior doors. Turn off all fans, heating, and air conditioning systems. Close the fireplace damper. Get your disaster supplies kit, and make sure the radio is working. Go to an interior room without windows that's above ground level. In the case of a chemical threat, an above-ground location is preferable because some chemicals are heavier than air, and may seep into basements even if the windows are closed. Using duct tape, seal all cracks around the door and any vents into the room. Keep listening to your radio or television until you are told all is safe or you are told to evacuate. Local officials may call for evacuation in specific areas at greatest risk in your community.

Another useful preparation includes learning some basic first aid. To enroll in a first aid and automated external defibrillator/cardiopulmonary resuscitation (AED/CPR) course, contact your local American Red Cross chapter. In an emergency situation, you need to tend to your own well-being first and then consider first aid for others immediately around you, including possibly assisting injured people to evacuate a building if necessary.

People who may have come into contact with a biological or chemical agent may need to go through a decontamination procedure and receive medical attention. Listen to the advice of local officials on the radio or television to determine what steps you will need to take to protect yourself and your family. As emergency services will likely be overwhelmed, only call 9-1-1 about life-threatening emergencies.

First Aid Primer

If you encounter someone who is injured, apply the emergency action steps: Check-Call-Care. Check the scene to make sure it is safe for you to approach. Then check the victim for unconsciousness and life-threatening conditions. Someone who has a life-threatening condition, such as not breathing or severe bleeding, requires immediate care by trained responders and may require treatment by medical professionals. Call out for help. There are some steps that you can take, however, to care for someone who is hurt, but whose injuries are not life threatening.

Control Bleeding

- Cover the wound with a dressing, and press firmly against the wound (direct pressure).
- Elevate the injured area above the level of the heart if you do not suspect that the victim has a broken bone.
- Cover the dressing with a roller bandage.
- If the bleeding does not stop:
    - Apply additional dressings and bandages.
    - Use a pressure point to squeeze the artery against the bone.
- Provide care for shock.

Care For Shock

- Keep the victim from getting chilled or overheated.
- Elevate the legs about 12 inches (if broken bones are not suspected).
- Do not give food or drink to the victim.

Tend Burns

- Stop the burning by cooling the burn with large amounts of water.
- Cover the burn with dry, clean dressings or cloth.

Care For Injuries To Muscles, Bones, And Joints

- Rest the injured part.
- Apply ice or a cold pack to control swelling and reduce pain.
- Avoid any movement or activity that causes pain.
- If you must move the victim because the scene is becoming unsafe, try to immobilize the injured part to keep it from moving.

Be Aware Of Biological/Radiological Exposure

- Listen to local radio and television reports for the most accurate information from responsible governmental and medical authorities on what's happening and what actions you will need to take.

Reduce Any Care Risks

The risk of getting a disease while giving first aid is extremely rare. However, to reduce the risk even further:

- Avoid direct contact with blood and other body fluids.
- Use protective equipment, such as disposable gloves and breathing barriers.
- Thoroughly wash your hands with soap and water immediately after giving care.

It is important to be prepared for an emergency and to know how to give emergency care.

✔ Quick Tip
More Information

All of these recommendations make good sense, regardless of the potential problem. For more information on how to get ready for disaster and be safe when disaster strikes, or to register for a first aid and AED/CPR course, please contact your local American Red Cross chapter. You can find it in your telephone directory under "American Red Cross" or through our home page at www.redcross.org under "your local chapter."

For information about your community's specific plans for response to disasters and other emergencies, contact your local office of emergency management. For more information about the specific effects of chemical or biological agents, the following websites may be helpful:

- Centers for Disease Control and Prevention: http://www.bt.cdc.gov
- U.S. Department of Energy: http://www.energy.gov
- U.S. Department of Health and Human Services: http://www.hhs.gov
- Federal Emergency Management Agency: http://www.rris.fema.gov
- Environmental Protection Agency: www.epa.gov/swercepp

Part Seven

If You Need More Information

Chapter 59

Resources For Information About First Aid And Medical Emergencies

American Academy of Neurology
1080 Montreal Avenue
St. Paul, MN 55116
Toll-Free: 800-879-1960
Phone: 612-695-1940
Fax: 651-695-2791
Website: http://www.aan.com
E-mail: web@aan.com

American Association of Poison Control Centers
515 King Street, Suite 510
Alexandria, VA 22314
Toll-Free: 800-222-1222
Phone: 703-894-1858
Fax: 703-683-2812
Website: http://www.aapcc.org

American Burn Association
625 North Michigan Avenue
Suite 2550
Chicago, IL 60611
Toll-Free: 800-548-2876
Phone: 312-642-9260
Fax: 312-642-9260
Website: http://www.ameriburn.org
E-mail: info@ameriburn.org

American College of Emergency Physicians
1125 Executive Circle
Irving, TX 75038-2522
Toll-Free: 800-798-1822
Phone: 972-550-0911
Fax: 972-580-2816
Website: http://www.acep.org
E-mail: sales@acep.org

About This Chapter: Information in this chapter was compiled from many sources deemed reliable. Inclusion does not constitute endorsement, and there is no implication associated with omission. All contact information was verified in July 2008.

American Public Health Association Injury Control and Emergency Services
800 I Street, NW
Washington, DC 20001-3710
Phone: 202-777-APHA (2742)
Fax: 202-777-2533
Website: http://www.apha.org/membergroups/sections/aphasections/icehs

American Red Cross National Headquarters
2025 E Street, NW
Washington, DC 20006
Toll-Free: 800-REDCROSS (733-2767)
Phone: 703-206-6000
Website: http://www.redcross.org

American Trauma Society
7611 South Osborne Road
Suite 202
Upper Marlboro, MD 20772
Toll-Free: 800-556-7890
Phone: 301-574-4300
Website: http://www.amtrauma.org
E-mail: info@amtrauma.org

Brain Injury Association of America
1608 Spring Hill Road, Suite 110
Vienna, VA 22182
Phone: 703-761-0750
Fax: 703-761-0755
Website: http://www.biausa.org

Burn and Shock Trauma Institute
Loyola University Medical Center
2160 South 1st Avenue
Maywood, IL 60153
Phone: 708-327-2446
Fax: 708-327-2813
Website: http://www.stritch.luc.edu/depts/bsti/index.html
E-mail: bsti@lumc.edu

Burn Survivors Online Inc.
Website: http://www.BurnSurvivorsOnline.com
E-mail: info@burnsurvivorsonline.com

Emergency Medical Services for Children
2550 University Avenue, West
Court International Bldg.
Suite 216 South
St. Paul, MN 55114
Toll-Free: 800-660-7022
Phone: 612-813-7749
Website: http://www.emscmn.org
E-mail: info@emscnrc.com

Emergency Nurses' Association Headquarters
915 Lee Street
Des Plaines, IL 60016-6569
Toll-Free: 800-900-9659
Phone: 847-460-4000
Fax: 847-460-4001
Website: http://www.ena.org
E-mail: enainfo@ena.org

Federal Highway Administration
U.S. Department of Transportation
1200 New Jersey Avenue, SE
Washington, DC 20590
Phone: 202-366-6836
Website: http://safety.fhwa.dot.gov

First Aid and Self-Care Guide
MayoClinic.com
Website: http://www.mayoclinic.com/findinformation/firstaidandselfcare/index.cfm

International Society for Traumatic Stress Studies
111 Deer Lake Road, Suite 100
Deerfield, IL 60015
Phone: 847-480-9028
Fax: 847-480-9282
Website: http://www.istss.org
E-mail: istss@istss.org

King County Emergency Services
Office of Emergency Management
3511 NE 2nd
Renton, WA 98056
Phone: 206-296-3830
Fax: 206-296-3838
TTY: 206-205-7516
Website: http://www.metrokc.gov/prepare
E-mail: ecc.kc@kingcounty.gov

National Association of Emergency Medical Technicians, Inc.
P.O. Box 1400
Clinton, MS 39060-1400
Toll-Free: 800-34-NAEMT (346-2368)
Phone: 601-924-7744
Fax: 601-924-7325
Website: http://www.naemt.org
E-mail: info@naemt.org

National Association of EMS Physicians
P.O. Box 15945-281
Lenexa, KS 66285-5945
Toll-Free: 800-228-3677
Phone: 913-492-5858
Fax: 913-541-0156
Website: http://www.naemsp.org
E-mail: info-naemsp@goAMP.com

National EMS Information System
P.O. Box 581289
Salt Lake City, UT 84158-1289
Website: http://www.nemsis.org

National Fire Protection Association
Phone: 617-770-3000
Fax: 617-770-0700
Website: http://www.nfpa.org
E-mail: nfparesfdn@nfpa.org

National Highway Traffic Safety Administration
1200 New Jersey Avenue, SE
West Building
Washington, DC 20590
Toll-Free: 888-327-4236
Website: http://www.nhtsa.gov

National Institute of General Medical Sciences
45 Center Drive MSC 6200
Bethesda, MD 20892-6200
Phone: 301-496-7301
Website: http://www.nigms.nih.gov

National Institute of Neurological Disorders and Stroke
P.O. Box 5801
Bethesda, MD 20892
Toll-Free: 800-352-9424
Phone: 301-496-5751
Fax: 301-402-2186
Website: http://www.ninds.nih.gov
E-mail: braininfo@ninds.nih.gov

National Safety Council
1121 Spring Lake Drive
Itasca, IL 60143-3201
Phone: 630-285-1121
Fax: 630-285-1315
Website: http://www.nsc.org
E-mail: info@nsc.org

National Strategy for Suicide Prevention
U.S. Department of Health and Human Services
Website: http://mentalhealth.samhsa.gov/suicideprevention

National Women's Health Information Center
Office on Women's Health
200 Independence Ave., SW
Room 712E
Washington, DC 20201
Toll-Free: 800-994-9662
Toll-Free TDD: 888-220-5446
Phone: 202-690-7650
Fax: 202-205-2631
Website: http://www.4woman.gov

Office of Emergency Medical Services
National Highway Traffic Safety Administration
1200 New Jersey Avenue, SE
West Building
Washington, DC 20590
Toll-Free: 888-327-4236
Website: http://www.nhtsa.gov/portal/site/nhtsa/menuitem.2a0771e91315babbbf30811060008a0c

Shock Society
Website: http://www.shocksociety.org
E-mail: webmaster@shocksociety.org

Shriners International Headquarters
2900 Rocky Point Dr.
Tampa, FL 33607-1460
Phone: 813-281-0300
Website: http://www.shrinershq.org

Society for Academic Emergency Medicine
901 Washington Avenue
Lansing, MI 48906-5137
Phone: 517-485-5484
Fax: 517-485-0801
Website: http://www.saem.org
E-mail: saem@saem.org

Society of Critical Care Medicine
500 Midway Drive
Mount Prospect, IL 60056
Phone: 847-827-6869
Fax: 847-827-6886
Website: http://www.sccm.org
E-mail: info@sccm.org

ThinkFirst National Injury Prevention Foundation
29W120 Butterfield Road
Suite 105
Warrenville, IL 60555
Toll-Free: 800-THINK-56 (844-6556)
Phone: 630-393-1400
Fax: 630-393-1402
Website: http://www.thinkfirst.org
E-mail: thinkfirst@thinkfirst.org

Trauma.org
Website: http://www.trauma.org

U.S. Fire Administration
16825 South Seton Avenue
Emmitsburg, MD 21727
Phone: 301-447-1000
Fax: 301-447-1346
Website: http://www.usfa.fema.gov
E-mail: usfaweb@fema.gov

Chapter 60

Resources For Information About Disaster Preparedness

American Association of Poison Control Centers
515 King Street, Suite 510
Alexandria, VA 22314
Toll-Free: 800-222-1222
Phone: 703-894-1858
Fax: 703-683-2812
Website: http://www.aapcc.org

American Red Cross National Headquarters
2025 E Street, NW
Washington, DC 20006
Toll-Free: 800-REDCROSS (733-2767)
Phone: 703-206-6000
Website: http://www.redcross.org

Boy Scouts of America
Emergency Preparedness Plan
Website: http://www.scouting.org/HealthandSafety/GSS/gss05.aspx

Center for Disability Issues and the Health Professions
Evacuation Preparedness Guide
Website: http://www.cdihp.org/evacuation/toc.html

Disaster Training International
9400 Ravenna Avenue, NE #7
Seattle, WA 98115
Phone: 206-420-8217
Website: http://www.disastertraining.org

About This Chapter: Information in this chapter was compiled from many sources deemed reliable. Inclusion does not constitute endorsement, and there is no implication associated with omission. All contact information was verified in July 2008.

Emergency Planning and Community Right-To-Know Act (EPCRA) Hotline
1200 Pennsylvania Avenue, NW
Washington, DC 20460
Toll-Free: 800-424-9346
Phone: 703-412-9810
TDD: 800-553-7672 or
703-412-3323
Website: http://www.epa.gov/epaoswer/hotline

Emergency Preparedness and Response
CDC, 1600 Clifton Road
Atlanta, GA 30333
Toll-Free: 800-CDC-INFO
(800-232-4636)
Website: http://emergency.cdc.gov
E-mail: cdcinfo@cdc.gov

Emergency Preparedness Tips
Website: http://www.emergencypreparednesstips.org

Federal Emergency Management Agency (FEMA)
500 C Street, SW
Washington, DC 20472
Toll-Free: 800-621-FEMA (3362)
Phone: 202-566-1600
Website: http://www.fema.gov
FEMA for Kids: http://www.fema.gov/kids

National Fire Protection Association
Phone: 617-770-3000
Fax: 617-770-0700
Website: http://www.nfpa.org
E-mail: nfparesfdn@nfpa.org

National Pesticide Information Center
Oregon State University
333 Weniger Hall
Corvallis, OR 97331-6502
Toll-Free: 800-858-7378
Website: http://npic.orst.edu
E-mail: npic@ace.orst.edu

National Safety Council
1121 Spring Lake Drive
Itasca, IL 60143-3201
Phone: 630-285-1121
Fax: 630-285-1315
Website: http://www.nsc.org
E-mail: info@nsc.org

Office of Air Quality Planning and Standards
109 TW Alexander Dr.
Durham, NC 27711
Phone: 919-541-5504
Fax: 919-541-1818
Website: http://www.epa.gov/oar/oaqps

Resources For Information About Disaster Preparedness

Preparedness Center
Website: http://www.prepared ness.com/asadvertised.html
E-mail: info@preparedness.com

Safe Drinking Water Hotline
U.S. Environmental Protection Agency
Hotline: 800-426-4791
E-mail: hotline-sdwa@epa.gov

Storet Water Quality System Hotline
U.S. Environmental Protection Agency
Hotline: 800-424-9067
Website: http://www.epa.gov/storet
E-mail: storet@epa.gov

U.S. Department of Homeland Security
Washington, DC 20528
Phone: 202-282-8010
Ready Kids: http://www.ready.gov/kids
E-mail: ready@dhs.gov

U.S. Environmental Protection Agency
Clean Air Markets Division
1200 Pennsylvania Avenue, NW
Mail Code 6204N
Washington, DC 20460
Phone: 202-343-9620
Website: http://www.epa.gov/acidrain/index.html

U.S. Fire Administration
16825 South Seton Avenue
Emmitsburg, MD 21727
Phone: 301-447-1000
Fax: 301-447-1346
Website: http://www.usfa.fema.gov
E-mail: usfaweb@fema.gov

Index

Index

Page numbers that appear in *Italics* refer to illustrations. Page numbers that have a small 'n' after the page number refer to information shown as Notes at the beginning of each chapter. Page numbers that appear in **Bold** refer to information contained in boxes on that page (except Notes information at the beginning of each chapter).

Numeric

"9-1-1 General Information" (National Emergency Number Association) 7n
911 calls
   chemical burns 378–79
   motor vehicle accidents 198–99
   overview 3–15, 7–15
   pranks **4**
   service charges **8**
   VoIP telephones **14**, **15**

A

AAA Foundation for Traffic Safety, headlight safety publication 161n
AAFP *see* American Academy of Family Physicians
ACEP *see* American College of Emergency Physicians
acids, chemical burns 80–81, **82**
A.D.A.M., Inc., substance abuse first aid publication 119n
Adams, W. Mark 11
age factor
   all-terrain vehicles 315–17

age factor, continued
   farm work **291**
   graduated driver licensing 136–37
   jobs **290**, 291, 293
aggressive driving
   coping strategies **194**
   described 131
   overview 193–96
air bags
   inflation process *148*
   on/off switches **146**
   overview 145–51
   safety belts **142**, **151**
alcohol abuse
   college campuses **181**
   death 122–24
alcohol use
   date rape drugs **223**
   motorcycle accident deaths 207–8, **208**
   motor vehicle accidents 128, 130, 196
   pedestrian safety 216
   snowmobile safety 319–20
   traumatic brain injury 110
   young drivers 179–84
allergies, insect stings 60
all-terrain vehicles (ATV), overview 315–17

"All-Terrain Vehicle (ATV) Safety" (National Safety Council) 315n
"All You Ever Wanted to Know about Fire Extinguishers" (Hanford Fire Department) 261n
"Always Expect a Train" (Federal Highway Administration) 211n
American Academy of Family Physicians (AAFP), publications
  animal bites 62n
  snake bites 65n
American Academy of Neurology, contact information 395
American Association of Poison Control Centers, contact information 395, 401
American Burn Association, contact information 395
American College of Emergency Physicians (ACEP), contact information 395
American National Red Cross, terrorism preparation publication 385n
American Public Health Association Injury Control and Emergency Services, contact information 396
American Red Cross
  chemical emergencies publication 369n
  National Headquarters
    contact information 396, 401
American Trauma Society, contact information 396
ammonia, chemical burns **82**
animal bites
  first aid **30**
  overview 62–67
  prevention **64**
apoptosis, research **100**
"Are You An Aggressive Driver?" (NHTSA) 189n
"Are You A Working Teen?" (NIOSH) 289n
arterial bleeding, described 20
artificial respiration, described 31–32
ATV *see* all-terrain vehicles
automobile safety
  aggressive driving 193–96
  air bags 145–51
  alcohol use 179–84
  bad weather 169–72

automobile safety, continued
  defensive driving 131–34
  drowsy driving 173–77
  drugged driving 185–88
  graduated driver licensing 135–40
  headlights 161–67
  inattentive driving 189–93
  night driving 161–67
  overview 127–30
  power outages 279–80
  safety belts 141–44
  tires 153–60
  winter storms 360–61
  see also motor vehicle accidents
avalanches, snowmobile safety **324**
avascular necrosis, described **91**
avulsion fracture, described 87

B

babysitting
  911 calls 5
  emergency information **245**
  expectations **247**
  overview 243–48
"Babysitting Basics" (Nemours Foundation) 243n
"Bad-Weather Driving" (Nemours Foundation) 169n
bases, chemical burns 80–81, **82**
"Basic First Aid Guidelines" (Muscogee [Creek] Nation Emergency Management) 17n
"Bedroom Fire Safety" (US Fire Administration) 249n
bedrooms, fire safety 251–52
bee stings 59–60
"Beware Boat Propellers" (USCG) 307n
Bianco, Carl 35n
bicycle safety, overview 303–6
biological attacks, national security 383
bleeding
  diseases **70**, **72**
  first aid 20–21
  treatment 69–73
"Blinded by the Light?" (AAA Foundation for Traffic Safety) 161n
blizzard warning, defined **360**
blood rule, described 73

Index

blue-white HID headlights **167**
boating safety, overview 307–13
Boy Scouts of America, website
  address 401
brain damage
  concussion **102**
  inhalation abuse **123**
  see also concussion; traumatic brain injury
"Brain Injuries and Mass Casualty Events"
  (CDC) 107n
Brain Injury Association of America,
  contact information 396
broken bones *see* fractures
"Broken Bones" (NHS Direct Online) 87n
bruises, first aid **30**
"Bug Bites and Stings" (Nemours
  Foundation) 57n
Burn and Shock Trauma Institute,
  contact information 396
burn depth, described **77**
burn extent described **77**
burn prevention, described **259**
burns
  classifications **76, 77**
  electrical current 275
  first aid 24–26, **30, 84–85**
  gasoline **78–79**
  overview 75–85
  see also chemical burns; electrical burns
Burn Survivors Online, Inc.,
  contact information 396

C

caffeine, drowsy driving **177**
calcium, bone health 90
campfire safety 253
candles safety 260
capillary bleeding, described 20
carbon dioxide fire extinguishers 262
carbon monoxide detectors 266, 270
carbon monoxide poisoning
  overview 265–67
  symptoms **267**
cardiopulmonary resuscitation (CPR)
  babysitting 245
  chemical poisoning 376
  choking 115
  drug overdose 121

cardiopulmonary resuscitation (CPR),
  continued
  first aid 28
  overview 31–33
"Cat and Dog Bites" (AAFP) 62n
CAT scan *see* computed axial tomography
  scan
CDC *see* Centers for Disease Control
  and Prevention
cell phones
  911 calls 9
  inattentive driving 191–93
Center for Disability Issues and the
  Health Professions, website address 401
Centers for Disease Control and
  Prevention (CDC), publications
  adolescent drivers 127n
  power outages 273n
  safety helmets 303n
  sheltering in place 349n
  traumatic brain injury 107n
  traumatic events 49n
  water safety 307n
chemical accidents
  lawn maintenance 287–88, **288**
  national security 383
  overview 369–79
  prevention **370**
  quick tips **379**
  sheltering in place 349–51, **374**
"Chemical Agents: Facts About
  Sheltering in Place" (CDC) 349n
chemical burns
  causes **82**
  described 80–85
  first aid 26, **84**
"Chemical Burns" (New Zealand
  Dermatological Society) 75n
"Chemical Emergencies" (American
  Red Cross) 369n
chest pains, first aid 26–27
child life specialists, hospitalizations 46
Children, Youth and Women's Health
  Service (South Australia), bleeding
  first aid publication 69n
choking
  alcohol abuse 122–24
  first aid 21–22
  overview 113–17

"Choking" (Nemours Foundation) 113n
choking game, described **116**
Christmas tree fire safety 260
circuit (electricity), defined **275**
closed fracture, described 23, 87
cold stress, power outages 278–79
college campuses, alcohol abuse **181**
color codes, threat conditions 381–82
comminuted fracture, described 23, 87
complicated fracture, described 88
compound fractures
    described 23, 87
    infections **91**
compression fracture, described 87
computed axial tomography scan
    (CAT scan; CT scan)
    bone fractures **89**
    concussion 104
    hospitalizations 46
concussion
    first aid **102**
    grades 103
    overview 101–5
    sports activities 300–301
"Concussions" (Nemours Foundation) 101n
conductor (electricity), defined **275**
convulsions, first aid 28–29
cooking fire safety 257–58, 267
"Cooking Fire Safety" (US Fire Administration) 249n
"Coping with a Traumatic Event" (CDC) 49n
"Countermeasures" (National Sleep Foundation) 173n
CPR *see* cardiopulmonary resuscitation
"CPR: A Real Lifesaver" (Nemours Foundation) 31n
crime prevention tips **232**
crisis hotlines, trauma **53**
"Crossing Advice for Pedestrians" (Federal Highway Administration) 211n
"Cruisin' without Bruisin'" (NHTSA) 203n
CT scan *see* computed axial tomography scan
current (electricity)
    defined **275**
    effects **276**

D

date rape, described **223**
date rape drugs, described **223**
"Dealing With An Emergency" (Nemours Foundation) 3n
debris entrapment, coping strategies **383**
debris flows, overview 366–67
defensive driving, overview 131–34
"Define Aggressive Driving" (NHTSA) 189n
depression, traumatic events 49–50
disaster kits
    chemical accidents 372–73
    terrorist attacks 386
    see also emergency kits; first aid kits
disaster plans
    basics **340**
    chemical accidents 372
    form *342–43*
    overview 339–47
    pets **344**
    supply kits **345**
    terrorism **392**
    terrorist attacks 385–86
Disaster Training International, contact information 401
displaced fracture, described 23
downers, described 120
driver education
    alcohol use 183
    graduated driver licensing 140
    motorcycles 204
    safety belts 141–44
driver licenses
    defensive driving 131–34
    graduated 135–40
    motorcycles 207
driving safety
    car phones **184**, **192**
    driver inattention **192**
drowsy driving
    caffeine **177**
    gender factor 184
    overview 173–77
    risk factors **176**
drug abuse
    defined **121**

Index

drug abuse, continued
  drivers 185–88
  overview 119–24
  "Drug Abuse First Aid" (A.D.A.M., Inc.) 119n

E

earthquakes
  described 363–65
  quick facts **365**
  "Earthquakes: Facts and Fiction" (FEMA) 363n
  "Earthquakes: Home Hazards Hunt" (FEMA) 363n
electrical burns
  described **27**, 275
  first aid **85**
electrical current
  effects **276**
  power outages 276–80
  safety considerations 273–75
electrical fire safety 256–57
"Electrical Fire Safety" (US Fire Administration) 249n
"Electrical Safety: Safety and Health for Electrical Trades, Student Manual" (NIOSH) 273n
electric shock
  described 273–75
  first aid **277**
emergencies
  911 calls 3–15
  babysitting 243–44
  cardiopulmonary resuscitation **33**
  disaster plans 339–47
  natural disasters **6**
  preparations 18–20
emergency departments
  hospitalizations 43–44
  interns **41**
  overview 35–41
  spider bites **61**
emergency kits
  contents **198**
  disaster plans 341–47, **345**
  disasters **280**
  see also disaster kits; first aid kits

Emergency Medical Services for Children, contact information 396
Emergency Nurses' Association Headquarters, contact information 397
Emergency Planning and Community Right-To-Know Act (EPCRA) Hotline, contact information 402
Emergency Preparedness and Response, contact information 402
emergency warning signs, described 17–18
emotional concerns
  hospital stays **47**
  traumatic events **51**
energized (electricity), defined **275**
epiglottis, described 114
epinephrine kits 60
"Escape Planning: Get Out Safely" (US Fire Administration) 249n
eschar, described 83
esophagus, described 113–14
estrogen, bone health 91
evacuations
  chemical accidents 374–75
  terrorist attacks 388
examination rooms, emergency departments 38
explosions, national security 382–83
"Exposing an Invisible Killer: The Dangers of Carbon Monoxide" (US Fire Administration) 265n
extension cord safety 252, 256, 257

F

"Facts about Alcohol Poisoning" (NIAAA) 119n
"Family Supply List" (US Department of Homeland Security) 339n
farm work
  age factor **291**, **293**
  hazardous occupations **292**
Federal Emergency Management Agency (FEMA)
  contact information 402
  publications
    earthquakes 363n
    floods 353n
    hurricanes 353n
    national security emergencies 381n

Federal Emergency Management Agency (FEMA)
  publications, continued
    thunderstorm safety 333n
    tornadoes 353n
    volcanoes 363n
    wildfires 363n
    winter storms 359n
Federal Highway Administration
  contact information 397
  pedestrian safety publication 211n
FEMA *see* Federal Emergency Management Agency
financial considerations
  emergency departments 38
  graduated driver licensing 140
firearm safety
  friends **237**
  overview 235–38
fire escape plans 249–51, 254, 256
fire extinguishers
  babysitting 245
  overview 261–63
  safety ratings **262**
fireplaces, safety tips 254
fire safety
  overview 249–60
  wildfires 368
"Fire Safety Beyond the City Limits" (US Fire Administration) 249n
fireworks safety 252–53
first aid
  basic procedures 30
  burns **84–85**
  chemical burns 377
  concussions **102**
  drug overdose 121
  electric shock **277**
  lightning injuries **336**
  overview 17–30, 390–91
  shock 20
  terrorism **392**
First Aid and Self-Care Guide, website address 397
"First Aid: Bleeding" (Children, Youth and Women's Health Service) 69n
first aid kits
  contents **19**
  described 18–19

first aid kits, continued
  disaster plans 345
  disasters **280**
  safety tips 6
  see also disaster kits; emergency kits
first degree burns, described 24
flash floods, driving safety **171**
flashflood warning, defined **358**
flashflood watch, defined **358**
flat tires, safety considerations **154–55**
floods 358
"Floods" (FEMA) 353n
flood warning, defined **358**
flood watch, defined **358**
Foss, Rob 182
fractures (broken bones)
  diagnosis 89
  first aid 23–24
  overview 87–91
freeze warning, defined **360**
freezing rain, defined **360**
"Frequently Asked Questions" (National Emergency Number Association) 7n
friends
  alcohol abuse **124**
  snowmobile safety 321
  social situations safety 224–25
  swimming 307
frost warning, defined **360**
"Fujita Pearson Tornado Scale" (FEMA) 353n
Fujita Pearson tornado scale, described **355**

G

gasoline burns, prevention **78–79**
gender factor
  choking game deaths **116**
  drowsy driving 184
  motor vehicle death rates **128**
  safety belt use 142
  traumatic brain injury **109**
genetic studies, spinal cord injury **100**
"Going to the Hospital" (Nemours Foundation) 43n
"Graduated Driver Licensing" (IIHS) 135n
graduated driver licensing, overview 135–40
ground (electricity), defined **275**

Index

gun safety
  friends **237**
  overview 235–38
"Gun Safety" (Nemours Foundation) 235n

H

"H2O Smarts" (CDC) 307n
hail storms, driving safety **170**
Halon fire extinguishers 262
hand signals, snowmobile safety **322**
Hanford Fire Department, fire extinguishers publication 261n
Hanson, David J. 179n
"Hard Facts about Helmets" (CDC) 303n
headlights
  alignment process **163**
  night driving 161–67
  rainy weather 172
hearing impairments, 911 calls 9–10
heat lightning, described 336
heat stress, power outages 278
hedge trimmer safety 286
Heimlich, Henry **115**
Heimlich maneuver
  babysitting 245
  choking 113
  described 22, 114–15
helmets *see* safety helmets
"High-Rise Residents" (US Fire Administration) 249n
holiday fire safety 259–60
"Holiday Fire Safety" (US Fire Administration) 249n
"Homeland Security Advisory System" (FEMA) 381n
home safety
  described 223–24
  gunshot injuries 236–37
  household chemicals 370–71
Home Safety Council, poison prevention publication 269n
hospitalizations, overview 43–47
  see also emergency departments
"How Emergency Rooms Work" (Bianco) 35n
huffing (slang) **123**

"Hurricane Classification" (FEMA) 353n
"Hurricanes" (FEMA) 353n
hurricanes, overview 355–56
hurricane warning, defined **357**
hurricane watch, defined **357**
hydrochloric acid, chemical burns **82**
hypothermia, power outages 278–79

I

IIHS *see* Insurance Institute for Highway Safety
impacted fracture, described 88
inattentive driving, overview 189–93
infections
  burn wounds 80
  compound fractures 87
inhalation abuse, described **123**
"Inline Skating" (National Safety Council) 325n
inline skating safety 325–28
insect bites/stings, overview 57–62
insect repellents 62
Insurance Institute for Highway Safety (IIHS), graduated driver licensing publication 135n
International Snowmobile Manufacturers Association, snowmobiling safety publication 319n
International Society for Traumatic Stress Studies, contact information 397
internet phone service, 911 calls 12–15
interns, described **41**

J

jet skiing, water safety 309–10
job safety, overview 289–94

K

"The Keys to Defensive Driving" (Nemours Foundation) 131n
"A Kid's Guide to Tornadoes and Preventing Disaster Damage" (FEMA) 353n
King County Emergency Services, contact information 397

L

landslides, overview **366–67**
lawn edger safety 282–86
"Lawn Maintenance Safety" (Texas AgriLife Extension Service) 273n
lawn maintenance safety, overview 281–88
leaf blower safety 286–87
"Life Jacket Wear" (USCG) 307n
life preservers, water safety 309–11
lightning safety 333–36
"Live Safely in Your Manufactured Home" (US Fire Administration) 249n
longitudinal fracture, described 87
Lyme disease 60

M

magnetic resonance imaging (MRI)
  bone fractures **89**
  concussion 104
  hospitalizations 46
manufactured home safety 255–56
marijuana abuse
  described 120
  statistics **188**
medical treatment, sports activities **301**
medications
  911 calls 5
  burn wounds 80
  concussion 104
  drugged driving 185–88
  fractures 24
  insect stings 60
  poison prevention 270–71, 370
  proper disposal methods **271**
mental health professionals, posttraumatic stress disorder 51
microwave ovens, safety tips **259**
mosquito bites 57–58
motorcycle safety
  overview 203–8
  statistics 196
motor vehicle accidents
  air bags 145–51
  drowsy driving 173–77
  drugged driving 186–87
  overview 197–202

motor vehicle accidents, continued
  power outages 279–80
  safety belts 141–44
  statistics 127–30, *136*, *138*
  traumatic brain injury 110
mouth to mouth resuscitation, described 32
MRI *see* magnetic resonance imaging
Muscogee (Creek) Nation Emergency Management, first aid publication 17n
myelin, defined **97**

N

National Association of Emergency Medical Technicians, Inc., contact information 397
National Association of EMS Physicians, contact information 397
National Crime Prevention Council
  contact information **232**
  police departments publication 231n
National Emergency Number Association, 911 information publication 7n
National EMS Information System, contact information 398
National Fire Protection Association, contact information 398, 402
National Highway Traffic Safety Administration (NHTSA)
  contact information 398
  publications
    air bags 145n
    motorcycle safety 203n
    pedestrian safety 211n
    safety belts 141n
    tire safety 153n
    unsafe driving behaviors 189n
National Institute for Occupational Safety and Health (NIOSH), publications
  electrical safety 273n
  workplace safety 289n
National Institute of General Medical Services, contact information 398
National Institute of Neurological Disorders and Stroke (NINDS)
  contact information 398
  spinal cord injury publication 93n
National Institute on Alcohol Abuse and Alcoholism (NIAAA), alcohol poisoning publication 119n

Index

National Institute on Drug Abuse (NIDA), drugged driving publication 185n
National Pesticide Information Center, contact information 402
National Safety Council
 contact information 398, 402
 publications
  all-terrain vehicle safety 315n
  bicycle safety 303n
  school bus safety 240n
  snow sports safety 325n
national security emergencies, overview 381–84
"National Security Emergencies: Things to Know" (FEMA) 381n
National Sleep Foundation, drowsy driving publication 173n
National Strategy for Suicide Prevention, contact information 398
National Women's Health Information Center (NWHIC)
 contact information 399
 publications
  safety concerns 219n
  school bus safety 239n
natural disasters, emergencies 6
Nemours Foundation, publications
 babysitting 243n
 bad weather driving safety 169n
 bites, stings 57n
 cardiopulmonary resuscitation 31n
 choking 113n
 concussions 101n
 defensive driving 131n
 emergencies 3n
 exercise safety 297n
 gun safety 235n
 hospitalizations 43n
 motor vehicle accidents 197n
 sports safety 297n
nerves, spinal cord 95–96
neutral (electricity), defined **275**
New Zealand Dermatological Society, burns publication 75n
NHS Direct Online, bone fractures publication 87n
NHTSA *see* National Highway Traffic Safety Administration

"NHTSA Policy and FAQs on Cellular Phone Use While Driving" (NHTSA) 189n
NIAAA *see* National Institute on Alcohol Abuse and Alcoholism
NIDA *see* National Institute on Drug Abuse
"NIDA InfoFacts: Drugged Driving" (NIDA) 185n
night driving
 graduated driver licensing 138–39
 overview 161–67
night driving glasses, described **167**
NINDS *see* National Institute of Neurological Disorders and Stroke
NIOSH *see* National Institute for Occupational Safety and Health
nitric acid, chemical burns **82**
nosebleeds 71–72
nuclear attacks, national security 384
nurses
 emergency departments 39
 hospitalizations 45
NWHIC *see* National Women's Health Information Center

O

oblique fracture, described 87
occupational safety, overview 289–94
Office of Air Quality Planning and Standards, contact information 402
Office of Emergency Medical Services, contact information 399
online relationships
 described **229**
 safety considerations 226–30
open fracture, described 23, 87
osteomyelitis, described **91**

P

pain management, sports activities 301
pass-out game (slang) **116**
pathological fracture, described 89
pedestrian safety
 overview 211–16
 quick tips **213**
pets, disaster plans 341

phosphates, chemical burns **82**
phosphoric acid, chemical burns **82**
physical therapy, spinal cord injury 99–100
physician assistants, emergency departments 39–40
physicians
    emergency departments 39
    hospitalizations 45
poison control centers
    911 calls 6, 7
    chemical accidents 375–76
    contact information 122, **379**
    poison prevention 269–71, 370
police departments, emergency calls 231–34
posttraumatic stress disorder (PTSD)
    described 50–51
    motor vehicle accidents 200
potassium hydroxide, chemical burns **82**
power outages safety 276–80
power tool safety, lawn maintenance 284–87
pranks, 911 calls **4, 8**
pregnancy, safety belts **150**
Preparedness Center, website address 403
propeller strikes 312–13
PSAP *see* public safety answering point
Pseudomonas 80
PTSD *see* posttraumatic stress disorder
public safety answering point (PSAP), described 10–11

R

rabies, described 64–65
radiological attacks, national security 384
railroad property, safety concerns **214**
railroad tracks, safety 212–14
rape, described **223**
recreation therapy, spinal cord injury 100
relationship safety, overview 219–22
rescue breathing, described 31–32
rescuer, cardiopulmonary resuscitation 31–32
residents, described **41**
Richter scale 363
riding mower safety 283–84
road rage, coping strategies **132**
Rollerblade, described **326**
rule of nines, burns **77**
rules
    bicycle safety 303–5
    blood 73
    snowmobile safety 321
    snow sports safety **331**
    sports activities 301–2
rural fire safety 255

S

sacral, defined **97**
"Safe Bicycling" (National Safety Council) 303n
Safe Drinking Water Hotline, contact information 403
Safe Kids Worldwide, all-terrain vehicle safety publication 316n
safety belts
    air bags **142, 151**
    described 149–50
    motor vehicle accidents 190
    overview 141–44
    pregnancy **150**
"Safety Belts and Older Teens - 2005 Report" (NHTSA) 141n
safety considerations
    911 calls 5–6
    instincts **225**
    motor vehicle following distance **134**
    relationships 219–22
safety devices, propellers **313**
"Safety Experts Remind Parents: No Children Under 16 on ATV's" (Safe Kids Worldwide) 316n
safety helmets
    bicycling 304–6
    facts **306**
    motorcycles 205, **205**, 208–9
    sports activities 297–98
"Safety: How to Be Safety Savvy" (NWHIC) 219n, 239n
scald prevention, described **259**
school bus safety
    overview 240–42
    street crossings **242**

Index

"School Bus Safety Rules" (National Safety Council) 240n
schools
  gunshot injuries 237–38
  sexual harassment 239–40
"School Violence: Tips for Coping with Stress" (CDC) 49n
seasonal fire safety 252–53
second degree burns, described 25
seizures, first aid 28–29
sheltering in place
  chemical accidents 374
  notification 351
  overview 349–51
  terrorism 389
shock
  drug overdose 121
  first aid 20
  see also electric shock
Shock Society, website address 399
Shriners International Headquarters, contact information 399
simple fracture, described 23, 87
skateboarding safety 328–29
"Skateboarding Safety Tips" (National Safety Council) 325n
"Ski and Snowboard Safety" (National Safety Council) 325n
skiing safety 329–31
sleet, defined 360
smoke alarms
  babysitting 245
  battery replacement 251
  fire safety 251
  manufactured home safety 255
"Smoke Alarms" (US Fire Administration) 249n
snake bites 65–67
"Snakebites: Reducing Your Risk" (AAFP) 65n
sniffing (slang) 123
snowboarding safety 329–31
snowmobile safety
  avalanches 324
  hand signals 322
  overview 319–24
"Snowmobiling Safety" (International Snowmobile Manufacturers Association) 319n

snow sports safety
  fall tips 329
  slope rules 331
social situations safety 224–25
Society for Academic Emergency Medicine, contact information 399
Society of Critical Care Medicine, contact information 399
sodium hydroxide, chemical burns 82
space monkey (slang) 116
speech impairments, 911 calls 9–10
speeding
  defined 195
  speed limits 196
spider bites 58–59
  described 59
  emergency departments 61
spinal cord injuries, overview 93–100
"Spinal Cord Injury: Hope Through Research" (NINDS) 93n
spinal injuries, described 24
spine, depicted 95
splints, fractures 24
sports activities, water safety 307–13
"Sports and Exercise Safety" (Nemours Foundation) 297n
sports equipment
  overview 297–99
  proper fit 299
SSD *see* sudden sniffing death
statistics
  alcohol use 179–82
  all-terrain vehicle deaths 317
  bicycle injuries 303
  carbon monoxide deaths 266
  carbon monoxide poisoning 265
  choking game deaths 116
  drugged driving 185–87, 188
  electrocution deaths 274
  graduated licensing 137
  helmets, motorcycles 205, 208–9
  lawn maintenance deaths 283
  marijuana use 187, 188
  motorcycle accident deaths 204
  motorcycle accidents 206–7
  motor vehicle accidents 127–30, 128, 129, 136, 138, 187, 197
  occupational injuries 289
  pedestrian fatalities 211, 213, 215, 216

statistics, continued
  safety belts 141–42
  school bus accidents 240, **240**
  traumatic brain injury 108–10, **109**
  tsunamis **358**
  wireless telephones **13**
stem cells, spinal cord injury **100**
"Stop Speeding Before It Stops You" (NHTSA) 189n
Storet Water Quality System Hotline, contact information 403
street crossing safety **242**
Streptococcus pyogenes 80
students
  alcohol use 179–82
  disaster plans 341
  emergency procedures **376**
  gun safety 237–38
  hospitalizations 47
  school violence 51–52
  street crossing safety **242**
  terrorist attacks 386–87
  trauma 52–53
substance abuse, driving safety **188**
sudden sniffing death (SSD) **123**
sulfuric acid, chemical burns **82**
"Summer Fire Safety" (US Fire Administration) 249n
sunglasses, night driving **167**
super driving, described 132–34
surgical procedures
  bone fractures **91**
  hospitalizations 46–47
suspicious activities
  described **234**
  police departments 232–34

T

"Talk It Out" (US Department of Homeland Security) 339n
TBI *see* traumatic brain injury
teaching hospitals, interns **41**
technicians, emergency departments 40
"Teen Drivers: Fact Sheet" (CDC) 127n
"Teen Unsafe Driving Behaviors: Focus Group Final Report" (NHTSA) 189n

"Terrorism - Preparing for the Unexpected" (American National Red Cross) 385n
terrorist attacks
  essential documents preservation **386**
  overview 385–92
  sheltering in place **389**
  threat levels 381–82
Texas AgriLife Extension Service, lawn maintenance safety publication 273n
thermal burns
  described 75–80
  first aid **84**
"Thermal Burns" (New Zealand Dermatological Society) 75n
"Things to Know: Earthquakes" (FEMA) 363n
"Things to Know: Hurricanes" (FEMA) 353n
"Things to Know: Tornadoes" (FEMA) 353n
"Things to Know: Tsunamis" (FEMA) 353n
"Things to Know: Volcanoes" (FEMA) 363n
"Things to Know: Winter Storms" (FEMA) 359n
ThinkFirst National Injury Prevention Foundation, contact information 399
"Think Safe Be Safe: Poison Prevention Tips" (Home Safety Council) 269n
third degree burns, described 25
threat conditions, described 381–82
"Thunderstorms" (FEMA) 333n
thunderstorms, requirements **334**
"Thunderstorms: If Someone Is Hit By Lightning" (FEMA) 333n
"Thunderstorms: Lightning Fact and Fiction" (FEMA) 333n
thunderstorms safety 333–36
"Thunderstorms: Things to Know" (FEMA) 333n
"Thunderstorms: What is Lightning" (FEMA) 333n
tick bites 58
tire pressure, overview **156**

Index

tire safety
 flats **154–55**
 motor vehicle accidents 201–2
 overview 153–60
 pressure overview **156**
 puncture repairs **158**
 rotation patterns *160*
"Tire Safety: Everything Rides on It" (NHTSA) 153n
tobacco use, fire safety **256**
"Tornadoes" (FEMA) 353n
tornados, overview 353–54
tornado warning, defined **354**
tornado watch, defined **354**
trachea, described 114
"Traffic Safety Facts: Motorcycles" (NHTSA) 203n
"Traffic Safety Facts: Pedestrians" (NHTSA) 211n
transverse fracture, described 87
Trauma.org, website address 399
traumatic brain injury (TBI)
 overview 107–11
 treatment **108**
traumatic events, overview 49–53
triage, emergency departments 37
"Tsunami" (FEMA) 353n
tsunami, overview 357–58

U

unconsciousness, first aid 29–30
undisplaced fracture, described 23
unit secretaries, emergency departments 40
uppers, described 119–20
USCG *see* US Coast Guard
US Coast Guard (USCG), water safety publication 307n
US Department of Homeland Security
 contact information 403
 disaster plans publication 339n
US Environmental Protection Agency, contact information 403
US Fire Administration
 contact information 400, 403
 publications
  carbon monoxide 265n
  fire safety 249n

V

venous bleeding, described 20
vertebrae
 depicted *95*
 described 94
violence
 reasons **221**
 school safety 240
vocational rehabilitation, spinal cord injury 100
voice over internet protocol (VoIP), 911 calls 12–15, **14**
volcano eruptions 365–68
"Volcanoes" (FEMA) 363n
voltage, defined **275**

W

walk-behind mower safety 282–83
warming up, sports activities 299–300
"Warning Signs" (National Sleep Foundation) 173n
wasp stings 59–60
water safety
 overview 307–13
 power outages 277–78
 quick tips **309**, **310**
 snowmobiles 323
weather
 driving tips 169–72
 earthquakes 363–65
 floods 358
 hurricanes 355–56
 lightning safety 333–36
 power outages 278–79
 sheltering in place 349–51
 tornados 353–54
 tsunami 357–58
 water safety 308
 winter storms 359–61
weather radio
 described **347**
Wechsler, Henry 181
weed trimmer safety 285
West Nile virus 57–58
"What Is Drowsy Driving?" (National Sleep Foundation) 173n

"What to Do after a Car Accident"
 (Nemours Foundation) 197n
"What to Do If There Is a Chemical and
 Biological Attack" (FEMA) 381n
"What to Do If There Is an Explosion"
 (FEMA) 381n
"What to Do If There Is a Nuclear or
 Radiological Attack" (FEMA) 381n
"What You Need to Know about Air Bags"
 (NHTSA) 145n
"When To Call The Police" (National
 Crime Prevention Council) 231n
"Who Is At Risk?" (National Sleep
 Foundation) 173n
"Wildfires" (FEMA) 363n
wildfires, described 368
winds, driving safety **172**
"Winter Fires: Safety Tips for the Home"
 (US Fire Administration) 249n
"Winter Storms" (FEMA) 359n
winter storms, overview 359–61
winter storm warning, defined **360**
winter storm watch, defined **360**
winter weather advisory, defined **360**
"Winter Weather Makes Driving More
 Difficult" (FEMA) 359n
"Wireless 9-1-1 Overview" (National
 Emergency Number Association) 7n
wireless 911 service, overview 10–12
wireless phones, 911 calls 9
wireless telephones, statistics **13**
withdrawal symptoms, drug abuse 120
wood stoves, safety tips **254**
wounds
 bleeding 69–73
 first aid 20–21, **30**
 spinal cord injuries 93

X

x-rays
 bone fractures **89**
 hospitalizations 46

Y

"Young Drivers and Alcohol" (Hanson)
 179n